Recent Results
in Cancer Research   146

Managing Editors
P. M. Schlag, Berlin · H.-J. Senn, St. Gallen

Associate Editors
V. Diehl, Cologne · D. M. Parkin, Lyon
M. F. Rajewsky, Essen · R. Rubens, London
M. Wannenmacher, Heidelberg

Founding Editor
P. Rentchnik, Geneva

Springer
*Berlin
Heidelberg
New York
Barcelona
Budapest
Hong Kong
London
Milan
Paris
Santa Clara
Singapore
Tokyo*

P. M. Schlag (Ed.)

Rectal Cancer
Surgical Management, Basic and Clinical Research

With 66 Figures, some in Color and 41 Tables

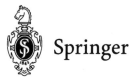 Springer

Prof. Dr. med. Peter M. Schlag
Klinik für Chirurgie und Chirurgische Onkologie
Universitätsklinikum Charité, Robert-Rössle-Klinik
Lindenberger Weg 80, D-13125 Berlin

ISBN-13: 978-3-642-71969-1 e-ISBN-13: 978-3-642-71967-7
DOI: 10.1007/978-3-642-71967-7
ISSN 0080-0015

Library of Congress Cataloging-in-Publication Data applied for
Rectal cancer: surgical management, basic and clinical research / P.M. Schlag (ed.). (Recent results in cancer research, ISSN 0080-0015; 146) Includes bibliographical references and index. 1. Rectum-Cancer. 2. Rec- tum-Cancer-Surgery.
I. Schlag, P.M. (Peter), 1948- . II. Series. [DNLM: 1. Rectal Neoplasms-surgery. W1 RE106P v. 146 1998 / WI 610 R312 1998] RC280.R35 vol. 146 [RC280.R37] 616.99'435-dc21 DNLM/DLC for Library of Congress

This work is subject to copyright. All rights are reserved, whether the whole or part of the material is concerned, specifically the rights of translation, reprinting, reuse of illustrations, recitation, broadcasting, reproduction on microfilm or in any other way, and storage in data banks. Duplication of this publication or parts thereof is permitted only under the provisions of the German Copyright Law of September 9, 1965, in its current version, and permission for use must always be obtained from Springer-Verlag. Violations are liable for prosecution under the German Copyright Law.

© Springer-Verlag Berlin · Heidelberg 1998
Softcover reprint of the hardcover 1st edition 1998

The use of general descriptive names, registered names, trademarks, etc. in this publication does not imply, even in the absence of a specific statement, that such names are exempt from the relevant protective laws and regulations and therefore free for general use.

Product liability: The publisher cannot guarantee the accuracy of any information about dosage and application contained in this book. In every individual case the user must check such information by consulting the relevant literature.

Production: PRO EDIT GmbH, Heidelberg
Typesetting: K+V Fotosatz GmbH, Beerfelden

SPIN 10568369   19/3133-5 4 3 2 1 0 – Printed on acid-free paper

Preface

Rectal cancer is an exceptional tumour entity within the variety of gastrointestinal tumours. While clinical techniques such as rectal digital examination and endoscopy would enable diagnosis as early as the stage of polypoid preneoplasia, only 10% of rectal cancer patients undergo surgery at an early stage of the disease. The prognosis of rectal cancer without infiltration of the muscularis is relatively good. However, with locally more advanced tumours, possibly associated with lymphnode metastases, the probability of successful treatment decreases considerably. Furthermore, there is a clear prognostic discrepancy between proximal and distal rectal cancers. Rectal carcinomas, especially in the distal location, except those diagnosed at an early stage, usually require surgical treatment with postoperatively disturbed or lost anal sphincter function. A permanent colostomy may not be avoidable. The current trends and developments in diagnosis and therapy of rectal cancers may be described as follows:
- The search for new diagnostic procedures and the attempt to define risk groups for which intensive preventive measures would be clearly successful. New insights may come from modern molecular biology or molecular genetics, especially with regard to hereditary colorectal carcinoma.
- A further increase in the rate of sphincter-preserving surgery without impairment of local tumour control or overall prognosis. New surgical techniques such as transsphincteric resection, but also various multimodal local treatment regimens, especially for low-risk tumours, are promising approaches. However, exact preoperative staging is an essential precondition for such procedures. Sphincter replacement or sphincter-simulating surgical treatments might be an alternative.
- The search for therapeutic improvement in locally advanced tumours. A reduction in the local recurrence rate should improve the patient's prognosis as a whole. This will be achieved by multimodal therapy concepts, focusing currently on preopera-

tive radiochemotherapy, sometimes in combination with hyperthermia.

This book constitutes a topical report on the above-mentioned themes and demonstrates current solutions. It is based upon an international expert conference and summarises the individual experiences of the participants as much as current general knowledge. The major aim of this work is to contribute to the ongoing discussion and to stimulate substantially further development in the field.

Berlin, April 1998 *P.M. Schlag*

Contents

Molecular Biology of Rectal Cancer

Molecular Pathology of Colorectal Cancer:
From Phenotype to Genotype 3
   M. Dietel

Familial and Hereditary Non-polyposis Colorectal Cancer:
Issues Relevant for Surgical Practice 20
   F. H. Menko, J. T. Wijnen, H. F. A. Vasen, R. H. Sijmons,
   P. M. Khan

Staging and Prognostic Markers

Use and Applications of MRI Techniques in the Diagnosis
and Staging of Rectal Lesions 35
   T. J. Vogl, W. Pegios, M. Hünerbein, M. G. Mack,
   P. M. Schlag, and R. Felix

The Value of Tumor Markers in Colorectal Cancer 48
   M. Hünerbein

Surgical Strategy

Possibilities of Extensive Surgery 59
   W. Hohenberger, K. E. Matzel, and U. Stadelmeier

Total Mesorectal Excision for Cancer of the Rectum 66
   P. Aeberhard and F. Fasolini

Radical Surgery for Extensive Rectal Cancer: Is It Worthwhile? 71
   F. L. Moffat, Jr., and R. E. Falk

Sphincter Preservation and Sphincter Reconstruction

Coloanal J-Pouch Reconstruction Following Low Rectal Resection .. 87
   K.-H. Fuchs, M. Sailer, M. Kraemer, and A. Thiede

Seromuscular Spiral Cuff Perineal Colostomy: An Alternative
to Abdominal Wall Colostomy After Abdominoperineal Excision
for Rectal Cancer 95
   P. M. Schlag, W. Slisow, and K. T. Moesta

Total Anorectal Reconstruction Supported
by Electrostimulated Gracilis Neosphincter 104
   E. Cavina, M. Seccia, and M. Chiarugi

Local Excision of Rectal Cancer Through Windowed Specula:
Long-Term Results 114
   W. Slisow, K. T. Moesta, and P. M. Schlag

Prevention of Local Recurrence

Locoregional Recurrence of Rectal Cancer:
Biological and Technical Aspects of Surgical Failure 127
   P. Hohenberger

Radiochemotherapy as an Adjuvant Treatment for Rectal Cancer .. 141
   L. Påhlman

Intraoperative Radiotherapy as Adjuvant Treatment
for Stage II/III Rectal Carcinoma 152
   M. J. Eble, T. Lehnert, C. Herfarth, and M. Wannenmacher

Radical Sphincter Preservation Surgery with Coloanal Anastomosis
Following High-Dose External Irradiation
for the Very Low Lying Rectal Cancer 161
   G. J. Marks, J. H. Marks, M. Mohiuddin, and L. Brady

Radiochemotherapy and Hyperthermia in the Treatment
of Rectal Cancer 175
   P. Wust, B. Rau, J. Gellermann, W. Pegios, J. Löffel,
   H. Riess, R. Felix, and P. M. Schlag

Future Strategies to Improve Results of Therapy

Dietary and Chemopreventive Strategies 195
   R. W. Owen

Diagnosis and Therapeutic Relevance of Micrometastases 214
   E. Holz, K. Pantel, and G. Riethmüller

Subject Index 219

List of Contributors*

Aeberhard, P.[66]
Brady, L.[161]
Cavina, E.[104]
Chiarugi, M.[104]
Dietel, M.[3]
Eble, M. J.[152]
Falk, R. E.[71]
Fasolini, F.[66]
Felix, R.[35, 175]
Fuchs, K.-H.[87]
Gellermann, J.[175]
Herfarth, C.[152]
Hohenberger, P.[127]
Hohenberger, W.[59]
Holz, E.[214]
Hünerbein, M.[35, 48]
Khan, P. M.[20]
Kraemer, M.[87]
Lehnert, T.[152]
Löffel, J.[175]
Mack, M. G.[35]
Marks, G. J.[161]
Marks, J. H.[161]
Matzel, K. E.[59]

Menko, F. H.[20]
Moesta, K. T.[95, 114]
Moffat, F. L. Jr.[71]
Mohiuddin, M.[161]
Owen, R. W.[195]
Påhlman, L.[141]
Pantel, K.[214]
Pegios, W.[35, 175]
Rau, B.[175]
Riess, H.[175]
Riethmüller, G.[214]
Sailer, M.[87]
Schlag, P. M.[35, 95, 114, 175]
Seccia, M.[104]
Sijmons, R. H.[20]
Slisow, W.[95, 114]
Stadelmeier, U.[59]
Thiede, A.[87]
Vasen, H. F. A.[20]
Vogl, T. J.[35]
Wannenmacher, M.[152]
Wijnen, J. T.[20]
Wust, P.[175]

* The address of the principal author is given on the first page of each contribution.
[1] Page on which contribution begins.

Molecular Biology of Rectal Cancer

Molecular Pathology of Colorectal Cancer: From Phenotype to Genotype

M. Dietel

Institute of Pathology, University Hospital Charité,
Humboldt University of Berlin, Schumannstrasse 20–21, 10117 Berlin, Germany

Introduction

In the West, colorectal cancer is the second most common cancer in males and the third among females, with about 180 000 new cases being diagnosed per year in Western Europe. The overall 5-year mortality rate is 50-60% after complete tumor removal (R0), whereas it is very poor after R1/2 resections. Once the tumor has metastazised, almost all therapeutic approaches – chemotherapy with cytostatic drugs, immunotherapy with monoclonal antibodies directed to surface (glyco-)proteins of the tumor cells, gene therapy with transduction of genes to stimulate antitumor inflammation or to reconstitute mutations, and several others – have proved to be of limited efficacy.

To improve the situation, better understanding of the molecular events leading to this aggressive type of tumor is needed. An increase in knowledge would open up a possibility of more specific therapies against the tumor and preventive measures directed at avoiding the onset of this type of cancer. The present paper focuses on new approaches to defining genetic alterations of the different stages of colorectal cancer and to link these to morphological features, which are still the "gold standard" of diagnosis and prognosis. Prognostic assessment influences decisions concerning the aggressiveness of treatment, in particular that of adjuvant or neoadjuvant chemotherapy, and thus must be as accurate and informative as possible.

Methods to Used – Problems to Face

Pathologists should be aware of several limitations when results derived by molecular and biological techniques are transferred directly to problems of surgical pathology. Many new insights into the pathogenesis of cancer have been created using cell lines that certainly do not represent the tumor biology as a whole: the cancer cells in relation to the mesenchyme, the blood vessels, and so on. Even at the cellular level, in vitro experiments presumably do not reflect the majority of the malignant epithelial cells present in solid tumors, mainly because of the appearance of many additional mutations dur-

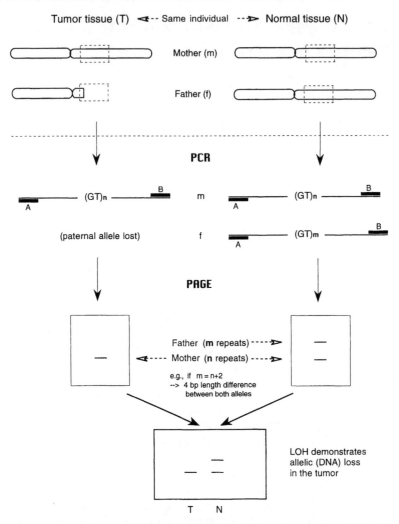

Fig. 1. One approach to molecular tumor characterization, PCR-based investigation of allelic DNA losses. This technique (for details see text) is known as detection of loss of heterozygosity

ing series passaging, and because of the selection of cells able to grow on plastic surface conditions. For all these reasons, data obtained experimentally should whenever possible be confirmed using fresh human material.

The techniques currently employed in molecular pathology include Southern and Northern blot hybridization, the polymerase chain reaction (PCR) and its variations such as reverse transcriptase PCR (RT-PCR), differential display RT-PCR (dd RT-PCR), as well as denaturing gradient gel electrophoresis and direct sequencing. These methods however, do not provide morphological information. It is possible for a portion of tumor tissue to be investigated, e.g., for point mutations or deletions, without confirmation that the tissue contains considerable amounts of tumor cells. In particular, this is likely in the case of stroma-rich tumors such as breast, prostate, colon, rectum or gastric cancer of the diffuse type, which may contain only a few malignant cells in the fragment selected for molecular analysis. Thus, results should always be interpreted alongside histological and/or immunohistochemical studies. Genomic abnormalities should be confirmed by in situ techniques, such as in situ hybridization (ISH), fluorescence in situ hybridization (FSH), or comparative genomic hybridization (see below). Similarly, RNA-based expression studies, e.g., Northern blot hybridization of tissue extracts, should be confirmed by sense/antisense ISH and, whenever possible, by immunohistochemistry to demonstrate that transcripts are indeed expressed.

The extent of genetic alteration suggested by any of the more global methods can be more precisely determined by loss of heterozygosity (LOH) analyses (Fig. 1), single-strand conformation polymorphism (SSCP), and direct sequencing. The latter has been facilitated by a new and simple nonradioactive technique for sequencing (Petersen et al. 1996). Since it is now possible to detect genetic alterations in some nanogram quantities of DNA, only very small tumor fragments are needed for molecular characterization. Hopefully all these approaches will add information on the possible behavior of a lesion and will lead to more accurate prognostication. The potential of molecular screening, e.g., using stool specimens from patients at risk of developing or already carrying precancerous or cancerous lesions of the colorectal region, remains to be evaluated rigorously.

In contrast to the above-mentioned molecular methods, which require considerable sequence information, a promising new method for a direct and global approach to the indentification of genetic alterations has been recently adopted by pathologists: comparative genomic hybridization (CGH). With CGH it is possible to screen the whole genome and gain a relatively precise overview of the losses and gains of DNA (for details of CGH, see below).

Histopathological Morphology: The Gold Standard to Be Beaten

All cancer staging systems seek to identify pathological features that may help in predicting outcome and may contribute directly or indirectly to guiding therapy (Table 1). The staging system used in colorectal cancer relies on the observation that tumorous lesions of the large intestine have characteristic morphological features that follow a diagnostic sequence of adenomas with mild, moderate, and severe dysplasia (grades I–III), or low-grade (mild and moderate) and high-grade dysplasia (Jass and Sobin 1989), leading eventually to frank adenocarninomas. The grade of a lesion's cytological and architectural dysplasia as determined by conventional histopathology is closely correlated to the risk of subsequent progression to colorectal cancer. This does not mean, however, that from the onset of malignant tumor growth the lesion is able to metastasize. The process of metastasizing only becomes rele-

Table 1. Independent prognostic factors of colorectal cancer

Factor to be estimated	Features	Importance for prognosis
Cytological grading	Grade I	Favorable
	Grade II	Favorable
	Grade III	Unfavorable
Architectural abnormalities	Low	Favorable
	Moderate	Favorable
	High	Unfavorable
R0 resection	Tumor margin not involved	Favorable
R1 resection	Tumor margin involved	Unfavorable
Tumor invades		
Lamina muscularis mucosa	pT is	No impairment
Submucosa	pT1 — see UICC	Only slight risk
Muscularis propria	pT2 — TNM classi-	Favorable
Through muscularis propria into subserosa	pT3 — fication	Unfavorable/poor
Other organs or perforates visceral peritoneum	pT4	Poor
Lymph node invasion	N0	Favorable
	N1 — see TNM	Favorable
	N2 — classification	Unfavorable
	N3	Poor
Vessel invasion	Histological evidence	Unfavorable
MIB1 determined proliferation		
DNA cytophotometry	Euploid	Favorable
	Non-euploid	Unfavorable
RAS gene mutations [a]	p21 level ⇧	Unfavorable
APC gene mutations [a]	Altered APC protein	Unfavorable
MCC gene mutations [a]	MCC gene product ⇩	Unfavorable
DCC gene mutations [a]	Adhesion protein ⇩	Unfavorable
p53 gene mutations [a]	p53 level ⇧	Unfavorable

⇧ increased; ⇩ decreased
[a] These results have been obtained by univariate analyses and need further confirmation

vant when the cancerous cells have been able to invade the mucosa through the lamina muscularis mucosae and enter the vasculature by which they become disseminated throughout the body. Since morphological ascertainment of these steps of progression by conventional histopathology is often difficult, it could be important to clarify whether the acquisition of metastatic potential is reflected in specific genotypic alterations. Because most of the patients die of distant metastases rather than of their primary tumors, defining a marker for this qualitative change would be undoubtedly highly relevant to pathological diagnosis.

The number of involved lymph nodes (20–30 nodes at least should be investigated by serial section histology), cytological tumor grade, invasion of blood vessels, degree of local invasiveness, and the presence of perforation and obstruction are further factors influencing the outcome of the disease and are often used as stratification factors in clinical trials (Galandiuk et al.

1992). More recently, in addition to these parameters, the proliferation fraction of colorectal cancer – i.e., the percentage of tumor cells engaged in mitotic cycling – has been investigated by several groups. When using the Ki-67 antibody or the new antibody MIB-1, which marks a formalin-resistant nuclear protein associated with the G1-M phase of mitosis, most groups were unable to establish its expression as an independent prognostic factor (Kubota et al. 1992; Diebold et al. 1994; Risio 1994). However, long-term follow-up studies with standardization of procedure are needed for a definitive verdict on the predictive value of the tumor growth fraction as determined by Ki-67 or MIB-1 (Sahin et al. 1994).

Identification of Metastases Indetectable by Histopathology

Micrometastases – especially in lymph nodes – may be missed by routine histopathological examination even when the tissue is processed and examined carefully. The possibility of detecting very small amounts of tumor-derived DNA or RNA – e.g., ras mutations, p53 mutations, or the RNA coding for cell-type-specific cytoskeletal proteins not present in normal lymph nodes – may significantly facilitate the detection of ever smaller metastases (Hayashi et al. 1994). Preliminary results show that in almost 30% of cases originally diagnosed as lymph-node-negative (N0), micrometastases could be found by molecular methods. This may become a potent prognostic marker and crucial in the decision to initiate adjuvant chemotherapy.

"Genetic Morphology": Screening of the Genome

Careful examinations of the clonal origin of epithelial mucosa cells revealed that the normal colonic mucosa is of polyclonal composition. An interesting fact, and one presumably of the utmost importance for understanding the monoclonality of mucosa tumors, is that the cells of any one mucosal crypt represent a clonal population originating from a single stem cell and thus are monoclonal. Since the cells of the adjacent crypt represent a "second" clone the mucosa in toto is polyclonal. A benign adenoma, even if showing only mild dysplasia, is found to be composed of monoclonal cells. This indicates that one cell acquired a proliferative advantage which may be a very early step towards unlimited growth. In addition, this observation confirms that monoclonality is not an unequivocal sign of malignancy.

In DNA cytophotometric studies of cellular dysplasia, the number of DNA hits was found to increase from grade I to grade III (Macartney and Camplejohn 1986). In colorectal cancer DNA aneuploidy was also found to correlate with advanced disease and with clinical outcome (Sun et al. 1993). Patients with an aneuploid tumor had a worse prognosis when compared to those with diploid tumors (Bosari et al. 1992), suggesting a direct relationship between the number of genetic alterations and the aggressiveness of the tu-

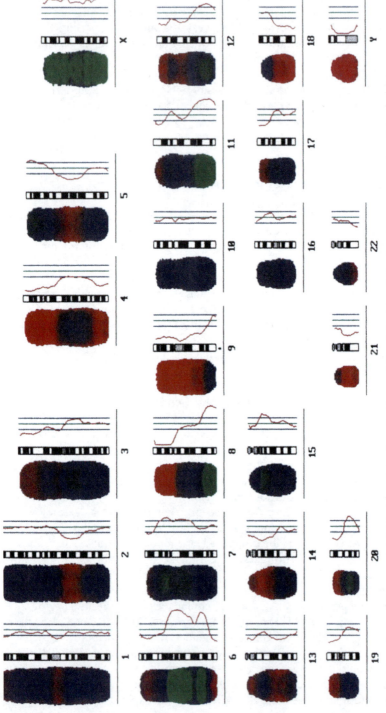

Fig. 2. A typical comparative genomic hybridization analysis of a colon cancer cell line. *Red* staining of the chromosomes represent loss of tumor DNA, *green* staining represents gain of tumor DNA, while *blue* staining is indicative of balanced amounts of DNA (blue is a software-born pseudo-staining instead of yellow in the preparations). The *vertical profile lines* demonstrate the ratio between gains and losses: *left of the midline*, loss of chromosomal material, *right*, gain of chromosomal material. *Note:* Chromosome 5q shows a loss in the APC and MCC gene region, chromosome 17p has acquired a loss in the TP53 segment, chromosome 18q is deleted in the DCC gene region, while the *mdr1* gene on 7q21 is overexpressed indicating multidrug resistance (the tumor expressed P-glycoprotein and was resistant to doxorubicin)

mors. In cases of regional lymph node involvement or distant metastases, DNA cytophotometry did not provide additional information.

Tumorigenesis in humans is associated with the accumulation of mutations in both oncogenes and suppressor genes. The steps of progression from an adenoma to a carcinoma are the result of an aggregation of multiple genetic alterations in the affected cells (Fearon and Vogelstein 1990). A new and promising approach to visualization of this accumulation of mutations is the method of comparative genomic hybridization (CGH). This can provide a genome-wide view of a tumor's complement genetic alterations (gene mapping) and thus may contribute to better understanding of the total number of DNA abnormalities (Ried et al. 1994). In brief, CGH uses a normal chromosome metaphase as matrix or standard DNA. To this matrix the total DNA of the tumor, labelled with a fluorescent marker, e.g., FITC, and the total DNA of normal tissue, labelled with another fluorochrome, e.g., rhodamine, are hybridized. The normal DNA preparation does not necessarily have to come from the tumor-bearing individual.

Hybridization with both tumor and constitutional DNA results in a metaphase chromosome stained in three possible ways:
(1) a mixture of red and green (→yellow), representing the situation that normal DNA and tumor DNA are present in the same amount;
(2) a green signal, indicating a gain of tumor DNA, i.e., an amplification; or:
(3) a red staining, showing loss of tumor DNA, i.e., deletions.

An example is given in Fig. 2. (Note: Balanced changes of chromosomes cannot be detected).

Initial studies in mammary and renal cell carcinmoma show that an increased number of genetic alterations correlates with poor prognosis (Isola et al. 1995; Moch et al. 1996). Several extended studies are currently on the way to confirm this and to increase our knowledge of the pattern of alterations.

Detailed Detection of Genetic Alterations

The most frequent genomic alterations described in colorectal cancer so far encompass chromosomes 5q, 17p, and 18p. It has been suggested that the biological properties of a tumor are influenced by the total number of changes and to a lesser extent by their sequence of occurrence, supporting the concept of a multistep process towards frank malignancy. Adenomas and carcinomas frequently show activating mutations in "dominant" oncogenes, such as members of the RAS gene family, and a combination of mutation and deletion affecting tumor suppressor genes such as APC, MCC, TP53, and DCC. Enhanced or reduced expression of the coded proteins promotes the malignant phenotype and appears to be associated with its malignant potential.

RAS Gene Family

Somatic alterations of the RAS gene family (H-ras, K-ras and N-ras) with overexpression of the ras protein, a 21-kD a protein with GTPase activity (p21), was found to be the most common (point) mutation in precancerous adenomas (grade III) and colorectal cancer. The mutations are not distributed randomly but appear mainly in the "hot spot" codons 12, 13, and 61. Immunohistochemistry detected p21 in about 50% in both grade-III adenomas and frank carcinomas, while low-grade adenomas (grades I and II) showed overexpression in only 10%–20%. Thus, altered p21 may be involved in the early stages of carcinogenesis. Ras genotyping clearly has prognostic value (Bell et al. 1993) and identifies patients whose colorectal cancer is more likely to follow an aggressive course (Sun et al. 1991; Finkelstein et al. 1993).

Immunohistochemical detection of the ras protein in tissue sections may be of predictive value in regard to the effectiveness of a new class of antitumor agents, the farnesyl transferase inhibitors. These drugs are able to interfere with the process of farnesylation of the ras protein precursor molecule, ras-GDP. Farnesylation is necessary for the activation of p21 and thus the ras-guided signalling process. Farnesyl transferase inhibitors are shown to inhibit or at least reduce the growth of epithelial tumors, as exemplified for experimental and spontaneous breast cancer in several animal models.

TP p53: The p53 Gene

Another important tumor suppressor gene in sporadic colorectal cancer was found on chromosome 17p13. The gene product is a 53-kD a nuclear phosphoprotein which in wild type has been shown to control check points of the cell cycle and regulate colonic mucosal growth.

Somatic mutations in the TP53 gene frequently lead to the synthesis of mutant proteins with a prolonged half-life detectable immunohistochemically. The mutated p53 accumulates in the cells and induces a dysregulated cell cycle with an advantage in cell growth. In accordance with Knudson's two-hit model, loss of one allele combined with a point mutation in the second occurs in 70%–80% of cases of colorectal cancer, while adenomas show a distinctly lower frequency when investigated by immunocytochemistry specific for mutated p53 (Tominaga et al. 1993). This correlation implies that the defect represents a relatively late event in the development of colorectal cancer.

Accumulation of p53 in colorectal carcinoma cells (Fig. 3) was shown to be an independent prognostic marker of overall survival and disease-free survival in several subsets of patients with colorectal cancer (Sun et al. 1992, Bosari et al. 1994, Hamelin et al. 1994). Monitoring of mutant p53 may be helpful in defining patients at high risk of recurrence who could benefit from a more aggressive therapy.

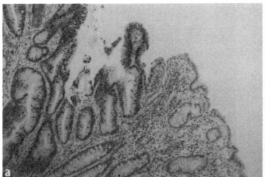
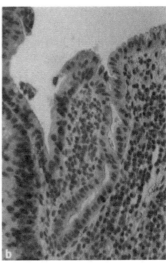

Fig. 3 a, b. Immunohistochemical demonstration of altered p53 overexpressed in rectal carcinoma cells. **a** There is a remarkably distinct border between the normal epithelial cells (*right*) and the p53-positive tumor cells (*left*). The stromal cells do not express p53 (×200). **b** Higher magnification of the zone of transformation (×630)

NME1/Nm23-H1 and NME2/Nm23-H2 Genes: The First Metastasis Suppressor Genes?

The closely related NME1/Nm23-H1 and NME2/Nm23-H2 genes have been suggested to be associated with a low frequency of metastases and to be metastasis suppressor genes. They are localized near the p53 locus, i.e, on chromosome 17q21. They were cloned by means of a murine melanoma model suggesting an antimetastatic effect for their respective gene products. While their sequence most closely resembles nucleoside diphosphate kinase, recent evidence suggests they act as DNA binding factors, increasing MYC gene transcription. In colorectal carcinomas, somatic allelic deletion involving 17q21 has been reported to be associated with the presence of distant metastases (Cohn et al. 1991) and more aggressive potential (Campo et al. 1994). However, it remains to be resolved how the NMEs' role of MYC activators can be reconciled with these results suggesting a tumor suppressor gene function.

These contradictions notwithstanding, cooperative alterations of the long and short arm of chromosome 17 eliminating TP53, the Nm23 locus, and possibly additional genes, may have further negative effects on the biological behavior of colorectal carcinomas.

APC (Adenomatous Polyposis Coli) Gene

By genetic analysis, the gene alterations responsible for the hereditary autosomal dominant disease of familial adenomatous polyposis (FAP) were localized to chromosome 5q21 (Groden et al. 1991; Kinzler et al. 1991a). This gene shows all the hallmarks of a tumor suppressor gene and when examined in sporadic colorectal cancer was found to be deleted in 60% of cases (Fig. 2). Interestingly, it was lost also in 60% of grade-III adenomas (Powell et al. 1992). Detailed analyses suggest that there is a further growth advantage when the mutation appears in both allele copies of the APC gene, but two mutations are not required for tumorigenesis. This indicates that mutations in the APC gene might be an important early step in colorectal tumor initiation. This view is supported by studies on the association of APC gene mutations and histological characteristics of colorectal adenomas (Benedetti et al. 1994; Jen et al. 1994a). When adenomas and hyperplastic polyps of the colonic mucosa were analyzed by SSCP, mutations in the APC gene were clearly associated with a more villous morphology, a growth pattern known to be prone to progression.

The APC gene product was found to be a cytoplasmic protein complex responsible for intracellular signal transduction from the zonula adherens reporting the state of cell-cell interactions. Mutated APC protein may deliver an abnormal signal, disturbing the regulation of cell growth and differentiation.

Patients with FAP and those with sporadic colorectal cancer suffer from similar or even identical molecular defects of the APC gene. Early detection of these mutations would be helpful in screening patients with respect to their risk of developing colorectal cancer. However, the wide distribution and mutational spectrum of this unusually large gene make mutation screening by conventional methods labor-intensive and costly. A novel approach using gel fractionation of in-vitro-synthesized proteins, the so-called protein truncation test, has increased the detection rate of germline APC mutations considerably (Powell et al. 1993), providing in 87% the possibility of molecular diagnosis of germline and sporadic mutations underlying this very common cancer.

MCC (Mutated in Colorectal Cancer) Gene

Another common region of genetic loss is found in a region closely physically linked to the APC gene, on chromosome 5q21-22. This is also suggested to be a tumor suppressor gene present in sporadic colorectal cancer and tumors associated with familial polyposis (Kinzler et al. 1991b). It encodes a protein with similarity to a G-protein-coupled m3 muscarinic acetylcholine receptor and may be involved in major cell signaling pathways controlling the cell cycle. Alternatively, the MCC protein has been speculated to be part of the complex structure of cytoplasmic intermediate filaments. It may be a kind of spacer that specifies distances between related filaments (Bourne 1991). Its dysfunction would create loss of organizational stability, giving these mutated cells an advantage in growth and presumably in motility – interesting ideas, but speculations that have yet to be proved. So far there exist no data on the relationship between MCC gene alterations and clinical outcome.

DCC (Deleted in Colon Cancer) Gene

Another gigantic gene spanning approximately 1.4 Mb has been localized to a region of the long arm of chromosome 18q, which is frequently lost in colorectal cancer (Fig. 2) and other advanced carcinomas (Vogelstein et al. 1988). The introduction of a wild-type chromosome 18q into human colon carcinoma cell lines resulted in flattened morphology and suppression of both anchorage independence and tumorigenicity in nude mice, suggesting a role in cell-cell contacts (Tanaka et al. 1991). Such a function is further supported by the DCC gene product's sequence similarity to the neural cell adhesion molecule N-CAM and other members of the cell adhesion protein superfamily. The DCC protein is expressed in normal colonic mucosa and has been reported to be absent in most colorectal cancers that have metastasized to the liver but present in the majority of nonmetastatic cancers (Zetter 1993). Allelic losses of chromosome 18q and reduction of the DCC protein correlate with decreased cell-cell interaction and attachment (Fearon et al. 1990). This may facilitate invasive growth and metastatic migration. Extensive studies on the association of allelic loss of chromosome 18q and prognosis revealed a role of this genetic alteration in tumor progression. The prognosis of stage II (Dukes stage B) cancer patients with LOH on 18q was similar to that of stage III patients, whereas stage II patients without 18q LOH showed survival rates similar to that of stage I patients (Jen et al. 1994b). If these results can be reproduced independently, they will provide a rationale for administering adjuvant chemotherapy based on 18q LOH status. All these results suggest that the DCC gene is another candidate tumor suppressor gene.

Since allelic deletion in chromosome 18q was also detected in adenomas, DCC alterations may also be involved as an early step of tumor development. Further studies on the role of DCC in normal and tumorous colon mucosa will provide information on the multiple functions of the DCC gene product.

MSH2/MLH1/PMS1/PMS2/GTBP: The Mutated Mutator Genes

Intensive research on bacteria have revealed a precisely working enzymatic DNA editing system controlling DNA replication and recombination through the detection of unpaired and mispaired bases. Mutations in these genes appear in 0.5% of the population and increase the risk of colon, ovarian, uterine, and kidney cancer as well as others.

In human colorectal cancer several genes, e.g., hMSH2, located on chromosome 2p22-21, and hMLH1, located on chromosome 3p21-23, have been discovered to be involved in mismatch repair. Recently, several studies investigating large kindreds with an excessive number of colorectal cancer patients have identified germ line mutations in a number of autosomal genes predisposing to syndromes of hereditary nonpolyposis colorectal cancers (HNPCC). Surprisingly, all five isolated so far show a strong similarity to previously known bacterial or yeast genes involved in DNA mismatch repair (Bronner et al. 1994). Somatic alteration of the wild-type allele by deletion or point mutation leads to defective proofreading of newly replicated DNA and thence to a greatly enhanced mutation rate in rapidly dividing tissues such as intestinal mucosa. Collectively, mutations in any of these DNA repair genes may well be the most important genetic predisposing factors in colorectal carcinogenesis. Tumors of patients with HNPCC have a tendency to mucinous differentiation and dextrocolic localization, but most characteristically display extensive length variation in short genomic repeat sequences. A similar albeit less dramatic replication error phenomenon (RER) or genomic instability has also been reported in a number of apparently sporadic cancers of various locations. Initial studies suggest a more benign behavior of sporadic colorectal cancers displaying the RER (Radman and Wagner 1993). The translation of this burgeoning field into the practise of molecular pathology poses formidable technical and conceptual problems but will undoubtedly provide a host of new molecular markers of great diagnostic and prognostic potential.

Cytostatic Drug Resistance: The *mdr*1 (Multidrug Resistance) Gene

Normal surface epithelial cells of the colon mucosa contain a relatively high amount of P-glycoprotein, a membrane-bound pump protein able to remove structurally and functionally unrelated drugs from inside the tumor cells to the extracellular environment (Fojo et al. 1987; Dietel 1996). The substrates for P-glycoprotein are mainly toxic chemical substances. Since epithelial tumor cells of colorectal origin preserve the expression of P-glycoprotein (Fig. 4), it is not surprising that a common quality of these adenocarcinomas is the almost complete resistance to various chemotherapeutic drugs – except a moderate sensitivity for the antimetabolite 5-fluorouracil. P-glycoprotein overexpression decreases the intracellular concentration of the chemotherapeutic agents, resulting in noneffectiveness, and confers on the tumor cells the multidrug resistant (MDR) phenotype. The drugs involved are anthracyclines, epidophyllotoxins, alkylating agents, anthraquinones, vinca alkaloids, etc. – the so-called MDR drugs. The ability to overexpress P-glycoprotein is found in approximately 80% of colorectal carcinomas. P-glycoprotein was found to be the product of the *mdr*1 gene (Gros et al. 1986) located on chromosome 7q21.1 (Callen et al. 1987). An amplification is shown in Fig. 2.

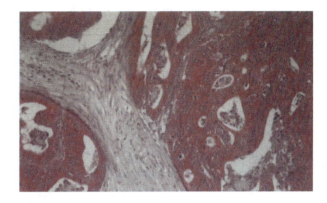

Fig. 4. Immunohistochemical detection of P-glycoprotein in an invasive adenocarcinoma of the rectum. Expression was concentrated not only at the cell membrane but was also detectable in the cytoplasm, indicating loss of polar differentiation. Clinically the tumor proved to be resistant to several chemotherapeutic strategies (×250)

Several approaches have been tested in vitro as well as in vivo to overcome multidrug resistance. Cell culture experiments revealed the strong potency of certain low-toxicity substances and antisense oligonucleotides to reverse multidrug resistance, e.g., verapamil (R- and L-form), cyclosporin A and H, PSC 833 (a cyclosporin derivative), dexniguldipine, anti-*mdr*1 ribozymes etc. (Juranka et al. 1989; Dietel et al. 1991; Holm et al. 1994). In animal models, too, MDR tumors were successfully modulated towards restored chemosensitivity (Dietel et al. 1996). in clinical trials, however, the breakthrough for the so-called chemomodulators has still to be established. The reason for this is certainly multifactorial and may be mainly based on the potential of the tumor cell to switch on differentially functioning mechanisms of resistance (Murran and Hait 1992).

In colon cancer, detection of the *mdr*1 gene in tissue specimens has been shown to correlate with local aggressiveness and prognosis (Weinstein et al. 1991). The same holds true for other tumor types. Whether this approach will reach diagnostic relevance remains an open question at present.

Telomeres and Telomerase Activity

The ends of normal human chromosomes comprise stretches of G-rich repeats. With increasing age there appears a reduction in average telomere length, an indicator of the number of cell divisions. Thus, physiological shortening of telomeres contributes to the control of balanced cell growth. Consequently, the enzyme which elongates telomeric DNA, i.e., the telomerase, is inactive in somatic cells in vitro and in vivo. Mutations of the telomerase genes, leading to upregulation or reactivation of the telomerase in tumor cells, may be an important if not essential event in the carcinogenesis of many tumor types.

In colorectal cancer, and even in grade III adenomas, the telomeric ends were found to be shortened (Hastie et al. 1990) or elongated (Schmitt et al. 1994) compared with the telomeres of normal mucosa. Independent of this observation, the telomerase appeared to be active and to hinder complete loss of the physiologic chromosomal ends. Since telomerase activity is detectable in colorectal carcinomas but not in simple polyps, it would appear to be associated with the acquisition of malignancy (Chadeneau et al. 1995). This of course results in prolonged cell life, giving these cells a growth advantage. No relation to clinical data is available on this interesting topic, but hopefully some will come soon.

Perspectives

A large number of sophisticated molecular techniques have become available which in combination with conventional histopathology, immunohistochemistry, and image analysis will increase the precision of the diagnostic workup of human tumor specimens. In colorectal cancer, molecular analyses of DNA alterations have already provided important insights into some mechanisms operative in dysregulated growth of the colonic mucosa. In addition, they may be helpful in evaluating the malignant potential of a given tumor and the likely clinical outcome under different therapeutic options. More studies are urgently needed to clarify whether the molecular approaches can provide us with information superior to conventional histopathology - especially for the individual case. At the present time, however, the diagnosis of colorectal cancer and the prediction of its biological behavior remain predominantly the task of routine conventional histopathology.

Acknowledgments. The author thanks Dr. Iver Petersen and Dr. Konrad Kölble, (both of the Institute of Pathology, Charité, Berlin) for their intensive discussion of the manuscript and their support with Fig. 1 and 2, and Gerti Stemmler for critical reading of the text.

References

Bell SM, Scott N, Cross D, Sagar P, Lewis FA, Blair GE, Taylor GP, Dixon MF, Quirke P (1993) Prognostic value of p53 overexpression and c-Ki-*ras* gene mutations in colorectal cancer. Gastroenterology 104:57-64

Benedetti LD, Sciallero S, Gismondi V, James R, Bafico A, Biticchi R, Masetti E, Bonelli L, Heouaine A, Picasso M, Groden J, Robertson M, Risio M, Caprilli R, Bruzzi P, White RL, Aste H, Santi L, Varesco L, Ferrara GB (1994) Association of APC gene mutations and histological characteristics of colorectal adenomas. Cancer Res 54:3553-3556

Bosari S, Lee AK, Wiley BD, Heatley GJ, Hamilton WM, Silverman ML (1992) DNA quantitation by image analysis of paraffin-embedded colorectal adenocarcinomas and its prognostic value. Mod Pathol 5:324-328

Bosari S, Viale G, Bossi P et al. (1994) Cytoplasmic accumulation of p53 protein: an independent prognostic indicator of colorectal adenocarcinomas. J Natl Cancer Inst 86:681-687

Bourne HR (1991) Consider the coiled coil. Nature 351:188-190

Callen DF, Baker E, Simmers RN, Seshadri R, Roninson IB (1987) Localization of the human multiple drug resistance gene, MDR1, to 7q21.1. Hum Genet 77:122-126

Bronner E, Baker S, Morrison P, Warren G, Smith L, Lecoe ML, Kane M, Earabino C, Lipford J, Lindblom A, Tannegard P, Bollag R, Godwin A, Ward D, Nordenskold M, Fishel R, Kolodner R, Liskay M (1994) Mutation in the DNA mismatch repair gene homologue hMLH 1 is associated with hereditary non-polyposis colon cancer. Nature 368:258-261

Campo E, Mique R, Jares P, Bosch F, Juan M, Leone A, Vives J, Cardesa A, Yague J (1994) Prognostic significance of the loss of heterozygosity of Nm23-H1 and p53 genes in human colorectal carcinomas. Cancer 73:2913-2921

Chadeneau C, Hay K, Hirte HW, Gallinger S, Bacchetti S (1995) Telomerase activity associated with acquisition of malignancy in human colorectal cancer. Cancer Res. 55:2533-2536

Cohn KH, Wang-FS, Desoto-LaPaix F, Solomon WB, Patterson LG, Arnold MR, Weimar J, Feldman JG, Levy-AT, Leone A (1991) Association of nm23-H1 allelic deletions with distant metastases. Lancet 338:722-724

Diebold J, Dopfer K, Lai M, Lohrs U (1994) Comparison of different monoclonal antibodies for the immunohistochemical assessment of cell proliferation in routine colorectal biopsy specimens. Scand J Gastroenterol 29:47-53

Dietel M (1991) What's new in cytostatic drug resistance. Pathol Res Pract 187:892-905

Dietel M (1996) Molecular mechanisms and possibilities of overcoming of drug resistance in gastrointestinal tumors. In: Kreuser P, Schlag P (eds) New perspectives in molecular and clinical management of gastroinstestinal tumors. (Recent results in cancer research, vol. 142) Springer, Berlin Heidelberg New York, pp 89-101

Dietel M, Boss H, Reymann A, Pest S, Seidel A (1996) In vivo reversibility of multidrug resistance by the MDR-modulator dexniguldipine (niguldipine derivative B859-35) and by verapamil. J Exp Ther Oncol 1:23-29

Fearon E, Cho K, Nigro J, Kern S, Simons J, Ruppert J, Hamilton S, Preisinger A, Thomas G, Kinzler K, Vogelstein B (1990) Identification of a chromosome 18q gene that is altered in colorectal cancer. Science 247:49-56

Fearon ER, Vogelstein B (1990) A genetic model of colorectal tumorigenesis. Cell 61:759-767

Finkelstein SD, Sayegh R, Christensen S, Swalsky PA (1993) Genotypic classification of colorectal adenocarcinoma. Biologic behavior correlates with K-ras-2 mutation type. Cancer 71:3827-3838

Fojo AT, Ueda K, Salmon DJ, Poplacl DG, Gottesmann MM, Pastan I (1987) Expression of a multidrug-resistance gene in human tumors and tissues. Proc Natl Acad Sci USA 84:265-269

Galandiuk S, Wieland HS, Moertel CG et al. (1992) Patterns of recurrence after curative resection of carcinoma of the colon and rectum. Surg Gynecol Obstet 174:27-32

Groden J, Thliveris A, Samowitz W, Carlson M, Gelbert L et al. (1991) Identification and characterization of the familial adenomatous polyposis coli gene. Cell 66:589-600

Gros P, Ben NY, Housman DE (1986) Isolation and expression of a complementary DNA that confers multidrug resistance. Nature (Lond) 323:728-731

Hamelin R, Laurent Puig P, Olschwang S, Jego N, Asselain B, Remvikos Y, Girodet J, Salmon RJ, Thomas G (1994) Association of p53 mutations with short survival in colorectal cancer. Gastroenterology 106:42-48

Hastie N, Dempster M, Dunlop M, Thompson A, Green D, Alshire R (1990) Telomere reduction in human colorectal carcinoma and with ageing. Nature 346:866-868

Hayashi N, Arakawa H, Nagase H, Yanagisawa A, Kato Y, Ohta H, Takano S, Ogawa M, Nakamura Y (1994) Genetic diagnosis identifies occult lymph node metastases undetectable by the histopathological method. Cancer Res 54:3853-3856

Holm PS, Dietel M, Scanlon K (1994) Reversion of multidrug resistance in the P-glycoprotein-positive human pancreatic cell line (EPP85-181RDB) by introduction of a hammerhead ribozyme. Br J Cancer 70:239-243

Isola JJ, Kallioniemi OP, Chu LW, Fuqua SAW, Hilsenbeck SG, Osborne CK, Waldmann FM (1995) Genetic aberrations detected by comparative genomic hybridization predict outcome in node-negative breast cancer. Am J Pathol 147:905-911

Jass JR, Sobin LH (eds) (1989) WHO - Histological typing of intestinal tumours. Springer, Berlin Heidelberg New York

Jen J, Powell SM, Papadopoulos N, Smith KJ, Hamilton SR, Vogelstein B, Kinzler KW (1994a) Molecular determinants of dysplasia in colorectal lesions. Cancer Res 54:5523–5526

Jen J, Kim H, Piantadosi S, Liu ZF, Levitt RC, Sistonen P, Kinzler KW, Vogelstein B, Hamilton SR (1994b) Allelic loss of chromosome 18q and prognosis in colorectal cancer. N Engl J Med 331:213–221

Juranka PF, Zastawny RL, Ling V (1989) P-Glycoprotein: multidrug-resistance and a superfamily of membrane-associated transport proteins. FASEB J 3:2583–2592

Kinzler K, Nilbert MC, Vogelstein B, Bryan TM, Levy DB et al. (1991a) Identification of a gene located at chromosome 5q that is mutated in colon cancer. Science 251:1366–1370

Kinzler K, Nilbert M, Su L, Vogelstein B, Bryan T et al. (1991b) Identification of FAP locus genes from chromosome 5q21. Science 253:661–665

Kubota Y, Petras RE, Easley KA, Bauer TW, Tubbs RR, Fazio VW (1992) Ki-67-determined growth fraction versus standard staging and grading parameters in colorectal carcinoma. A multivariate analysis. Cancer 70:2602–2609

Macartney JC, Camplejohn RS (1986) DNA flow cytometry of histological material from dysplastic lesions of human gastric mucosa. J Pathol 150:113–118

Moch H, Presti JC, Sauter G, Buchholz N, Jordan P, Mihatsch MJ, Waldmann M (1996) Genetic aberrations detected by comparative genomic hybridization are associated with clinical outcome in renal cell carcinoma. Cancer Res 56:27–30

Murren JR, Hait WN (1992) Why haven't we cured multidrug resistant tumors. Oncol Res 4:1–6

Petersen I, Ohgaki H, Ludeke B, Kleihues P (1994) Direct DNA sequencing following SSCP analysis. Anal Biochem 218:478–479

Petersen I, Reichel M, Dietel M (1996) Use of non-radioactive detection in SSCP, direct DNA sequencing and LOH analysis. J Clin Pathol Mol Pathol 49:118–121

Powell S, Zilz N, Beazer-Barcly Y, Bryan T, Hamilton S, Thibodeau S, Vogelstein B, Kinzler K (1992) APC mutations occur early during colorectal tumorigeneses. Nature 359:235–237

Powell SM, Petersen GM, Krush AJ, Booker S, Jen J, Giardiello FM, Hamilton SR, Vogelstein B, Kinzler KW (1993) Molecular diagnosis of familial adenomatous polyposis. N Engl J Med 329:1982–1987

Radman M, Wagner P (1993) Missing mismatch repair. Nature 366:722

Ried T, Petersen I, Holtgreve-Grez H, Speicher MR, Schrock E, du-Manoir S, Cremer T (1994) Mapping of multiple DNA gains and losses in primary small cell lung carcinomas by comparative genomic hybridization. Cancer Res 54:1801–1806

Risio M (1994) Methodological aspects of using immunohistochemical cell proliferation biomarkers in colorectal carcinoma chemoprevention. J Cell Biochem (Suppl) 19:61–67

Sahin AA, Ro JY, Brown RW, Ordonez NG, Cleary KR, el-Naggar AK, Wilson P, Ayala AG (1994) Assessment of Ki-67-derived tumor proliferative activity in colorectal adenocarcinomas. Mod Pathol 7:17–22

Schmitt H, Blin N, Zankl H, Scherthan H (1994) Telomere length variation in normal and malignant human tissues. Genes Chromosom Cancer 11:171–177

Sun XF, Wingren S, Carstensen JM, Stal O, Hatschek T, Boeryd B, Nordenskjold B, Zhang H (1991) Ras p21 expression in relation to DNA ploidy, S-phase fraction and prognosis in colorectal adenocarcinoma. Eur J Cancer 27:1646–1649

Sun XF, Carstensen JM, Zhang H, Stal O, Wingren S, Hatschek T, Nordenskjold B (1992) Prognostic significance of cytoplasmic p53 oncoprotein in colorectal adenocarcinoma. Lancet 340:1369–1373

Sun XF, Carstensen JM, Stal O, Zhang H, Nusson E, Sjodahl R, Nordenskjold B (1993) Prognostic significance of p53 expression in relation to DNA ploidy in colorectal adenocarcinoma. Virchows Arch A Pathol Anat Histopathol 423:443–448

Tanaka K, Oshimura M, Kikuchi R, Seki M, Hayashi T, Miyaki M (1991) Suppression of tumorigenicity in human colon carcinoma cells by introduction of normal chromosome 5 or 18. Nature 349:340–342

Tominaga O, Hamelin R, Trouvat V, Salmon RJ, Lesec G, Thomas G, Remvikos Y (1993) Frequently elevated content of immunochemically defined wild-type p53 protein in colorectal adenomas. Oncogene 8:2653–2658

Vogelstein B, Fearon ER, Hamilton SR, Kern SE, Preisinger AC, Leppert M, Nakamura Y, White R, Smits AM, Bos JL (1988) Genetic alterations during colorectal-tumor development. N Engl J Med 319:525–532

Weinstein RS, Jakate SM, Dominguez JM, Lebovitz MD, Koukoulis GK, Kuszak JR, Klusens LF, Grogan TM, Saclarides TJ, Roninson IB et al. (1991) Relationship of the expression of the multidrug resistance gene product (P-glycoprotein) in human colon carcinoma to local tumor aggressiveness and lymph node metastasis. Cancer Res 51:2720–2726

Zetter BR (1993) Adhesion molecules in tumor metastasis. Semin Cancer Biol 4:219–229

Familial and Hereditary Non-polyposis Colorectal Cancer: Issues Relevant for Surgical Practice

F. H. Menko[1], J. T. Wijnen[2], H. F. A. Vasen[3], R. H. Sijmons[4], and P. Meera Khan[2]

[1] Department of Clinical Genetics, University Hospital Vrije Universiteit,
P.O. Box 7057, 1007 MB Amsterdam, The Netherlands
[2] Department of Human Genetics, Medical Genetics Center,
Sylvius Laboratories, Leiden University, Leiden, The Netherlands
3 Foundation for the Detection of Hereditary Tumours, Leiden, The Netherlands
4 Department of Medical Genetics, Faculty of Medicine, University of Groningen, Groningen, The Netherlands

Abstract

About 15% of patients with colorectal cancer report a family history of this disease. An estimated 1%–5% of patients have hereditary non-polyposis colorectal cancer (HNPCC). Recently, DNA mismatch repair genes associated with this syndrome were identified. For about 50% of families in which HNPCC occurs, DNA-based diagnosis and presymptomatic DNA testing are now feasible. Diagnosis of a hereditary tumour syndrome is relevant for both the patient with cancer and his or her close relatives. The complexities of family studies warrant the forming of a multidisciplinary team which may choose to work within a specialized cancer family clinic.

Introduction

In recent years data on the genetic background of colorectal cancer have become available. A series of studies has revealed how genetic changes accumulate during the development of a colorectal tumour, i.e. during the progression from initial adenoma formation to malignant disease. In the future, these findings may have clinical importance, since the prognosis of the disease seems to be related to specific genetic alterations in the cancer cells (Shibata et al. 1996).

While all patients with colorectal cancer exhibit genetic defects in their neoplastic cells, a subgroup of patients also have a hereditary predisposition to tumour formation. These patients harbour a gene mutation in all body cells, a constitutional or germline mutation, which constitutes the genetic predisposition for cancer. Hereditary colorectal cancer usually follows an autosomal dominant pattern of inheritance: the gene defect is transmitted from one generation to the next with a 50% chance that the offspring of patients will inherit the cancer susceptibility.

From a clinical point of view patients with colorectal cancer can be separated into two main subgroups: sporadic patients, whose family history is negative for colorectal cancer, and patients with a positive family history. The latter group, which constitutes about 15% of cases, is characterized by occurrence of the disease in one or more first-degree relatives, i.e. a parent, brother, sister or child. In more than two-thirds of these familial cases the cause of familial clustering of colorectal cancer cannot be established with certainty. It may be chance, common genetic susceptibility, common exposure to harmful environmental (dietary) factors or a combination of these factors. Less than one-third of familial cases have a demonstrated hereditary origin. About 1%–5% of patients with large bowel cancer have hereditary non-polyposis colorectal cancer (HNPCC), and about 1% have familial adenomatous polyposis (FAP).

In this chapter several aspects of the genetics of colorectal cancer which are important in surgical practice are considered: familial occurrence of the disease, risk counselling for relatives of patients, possibilities of DNA-based diagnosis, the role of genetic predisposition in sporadic (non-familial) cases and management decisions for patients and their relatives. Illustrative case histories are presented.

Although cancer of the rectum differs from cancer of the colon in several respects (epidemiology, natural history, treatment) in this chapter they will be considered as a single entity called colorectal cancer. Only non-polyposis forms of large bowel cancer in which the patient has one or a few premalignant adenomatous polyps will be discussed. Polyposis forms of colorectal cancer, notably familial adenomatous polyposis, will not be considered.

HNPCC: Clinical Diagnosis

Diagnosing HNPCC is difficult because patients with this condition have no specific clinical features to distinguish them from patients with sporadic disease. The clinical diagnosis of HNPCC is based upon a family study in which occurrence of colorectal cancer in successive generations is demonstrated.

As a group, however, patients with HNPCC have certain features in common. Characteristically they exhibit early onset of disease (mean age at diagnosis of colorectal cancer in a Dutch series of 194 patients from 41 families: 44 years, range 16–74 years), tumour location in the proximal part of the colon (58% of cancers) and multiple primary tumour sites (23%) (Vasen et al. 1994).

Patients with HNPCC may also present with extracolonic malignancies. Endometrial cancer is by far the most frequent extracolonic malignancy associated with this syndrome. Other tumour types which fall within the spectrum of HNPCC include cancer of the stomach, small intestine, upper urological tract (renal pelvis and ureter), ovary and skin (Muir-Torre syndrome) (Watson and Lynch 1993; Watson et al. 1994; Hall et al. 1994a).

HNPCC follows an autosomal dominant inheritance pattern. Penetrance (the percentage of gene carriers who exhibit colorectal cancer or an extracolonic tumour) is about 90%. Initially, two subtypes of HNPCC were distinguished, one without and one with extracolonic tumours (Lynch syndromes I and II, respectively). However, it is now believed that this subdivision is invalid (Watson and Lynch, 1993).

The question has arisen how diagnostic criteria for HNPCC should be defined.

In 1990 at a meeting held in Amsterdam, the International Collaborative Group on HNPCC proposed the following minimal criteria (the Amsterdam criteria) for inclusion of families in collaborative studies:
1) histologically confirmed colorectal cancer in at least three relatives, one patient being a first-degree relative of the other two,
2) occurrence of disease in at least two successive generations,
3) age at diagnosis under 50 years for at least one patient; and
4) exclusion of familial adenomatous polyposis (Vasen et al. 1991).

However, these criteria have well-recognized limitations. A diagnosis might be missed if one were to adhere strictly to the Amsterdam criteria for diagnostic purposes, in particular since they do not include extracolonic tumours (Lynch et al. 1993; Menko et al. 1994). In general, therefore, the diagnosis of HNPCC should not be considered as established until an extensive family study and verification of the family history by means of objective data have been completed as far as possible. In large families with many affected individuals the diagnosis may be straightforward. On the other hand, in small families with only a few affected individuals the clinical diagnosis of HNPCC must often remain tentative.

HNPCC: DNA-Based Diagnosis

Only recently, in 1993 and 1994, has the genetic background of HNPCC been clarified. Apparently, HNPCC is a genetically heterogeneous condition, different genes being involved in different families. Five genes associated with HNPCC have now been identified. These genes normally have a function in DNA mismatch repair, which involves the identification and repair of base-pair anomalies that may occur during DNA replication. In most HNPCC kindreds a mutation of either the hMSH2 gene on chromosome 2 or the hMLH1 gene on chromosome 3 is involved (Fishel et al. 1993; Leach et al. 1993; Nicolaides et al. 1994; Papadopoulos et al. 1994; Miyaki et al. 1997). Most of the colorectal cancers in HNPCC families exhibit a characteristic pattern of widespread genetic alterations, the microsatellite instability (MSI) or replication-error-positive (RER+) phenotype, which is found in only a minority of patients with sporadic large bowel cancer (Aaltonen et al. 1993). Thus, HNPCC appears to be due basically to a disturbance of DNA mismatch repair which leads to genetic instability of somatic cells. This genetic instability is reflected in typical genetic alterations of the tumour cells, the MSI phenomenon. Examination of carcinomas for MSI has become of diagnostic importance in the evaluation of families for the presence of HNPCC (Jass et al. 1995/1996).

As a result of the discovery of involvement of the hMSH2 and hMLH1 genes in HNPCC, DNA-based diagnosis and presymptomatic DNA testing are now available to these families. In about 50% of HNPCC families which fulfill the Amsterdam criteria DNA studies reveal a defect in one of the mismatch repair genes. In a series of 86 unrelated HNPCC families the percentages of families with a pathogenic hMSH2 or hMLH1 mutation were 20% and 29%, respectively (Wijnen et al. 1995/1996/1997).

Clinical application of DNA-based diagnosis has now been described by several groups (van de Water 1994; Menko et al. 1996). One advantage of clinical application is obvious. Without DNA testing all children of HNPCC patients are advised to undergo lifelong periodic screening since their chance of inheriting the gene defect is 50%. For families in which the underlying gene mutation has been detected DNA testing will clarify who in fact is and who is not a gene carrier. For the latter group screening can be discontinued.

As a rule children are not subjected to DNA testing unless diagnosis will bring a medical benefit at a young age. In the case of HNPCC, preventive measures are not recommended before the age of 20-25 years, and therefore DNA testing is generally not performed until the children are over 18 years of age.

HNPCC: Management of Patients and Family Members

The biology of HNPCC differs from that of sporadic colorectal cancer. In both groups cancer originates from an adenomatous polyp. However, in HNPCC, premalignant adenomas are probably more likely to undergo malignant change than adenomas from patients with sporadic disease (Jass and Stewart 1992; Jass 1995). The observation of interval cancer (patients who present with symptoms in between colonoscopies) emphasizes the need for frequent examination of individuals at high risk of HNPCC (Lanspa et al. 1994; Vasen et al. 1995). Present data indicate that screening and polypectomy indeed reduces the incidence of colorectal cancer in this group (Järvinen et al. 1995).

For family members at high risk of HNPCC, many authors advise colonoscopy every 1-2 years from the age of 20-25 years. In addition, annual gynaecological screening from the age of 30-35 years is advised for all proven female gene carriers and for all women in whose family endometrial cancer has been observed. Screening for other extracolonic tumours is usually considered only if tumours that belong to the HNPCC spectrum have been observed in the family under investigation and if screening for that tumour type is feasible.

The high risk of a second colorectal tumour in HNPCC has led to a recommendation for subtotal colectomy as treatment in HNPCC patients with colonic cancer (Mecklin and Järvinen 1993). Because of the high prevalence of endometrial cancer in gene carriers (Watson et al. 1994; Vasen et al. 1996) the option of prophylactic hysterectomy and oophorectomy at the time of

Table 1. Management options for families with hereditary non-polyposis colorectal cancer (HNPCC)

At-risk family member:
1. Colonoscopy from age 20–25 years[a] every 1–2 years
2. For females: annual gynaecological examination from age 30–35 years if endometrial cancer is observed in the family
3. Screening for other tumours[b]
Proven gene carrier
1. See management for at-risk family member (above); * prophylactic colectomy
2. For females: annual gynaecological examination
3. Screening for other tumours[b]
Patient with colonic cancer
1. Subtotal colectomy
2. * For females: prophylactic hysterectomy and oophorectomy

* Optional
[a] Or 5 years earlier than the age of the youngest patient in a given family, if this yields an age less than 20–25 years.
[b] If other HNPCC-associated tumours are encountered in the family, and if screening for that tumour type is feasible.

surgery should be considered for females from HNPCC kindreds who present with large bowel cancer.

Since the advent of presymptomatic DNA-based diagnosis, the question has arisen whether proven gene carriers, who run about an 80% lifetime risk of developing colorectal cancer, should be subjected to prophylactic surgery. Prophylactic colectomy should be considered in particular if the individual has recurrent adenomas with unfavourable histological characteristics (Rodríguez-Bigas 1996).

The clinical expression of HNPCC varies markedly between and within families. Two potential determinants of expression are modifier genes (other genetic factors which influence expression of the gene mutation) and environmental (dietary) factors. Although dietary factors are important in the pathogenesis of sporadic colorectal cancer, it is not known whether these factors play a role in the expression of HNPCC. Therefore, dietary advice for the latter group is optional.

Since no clear genotype-phenotype correlations have as yet been detected for HNPCC, recommendations for management are at present independent of the gene or mutation identified in the family under investigation.

Management options for HNPCC are summarized in Table 1.

Familial and Sporadic Colorectal Cancer

Colorectal cancer occurs more often in relatives of patients than can be attributed to chance. However, in most cases the cause of familial clustering of the disease cannot be established with certainty. For example, two brothers are affected with large bowel cancer and no other family members have this condition or any other malignancy. There are three possible explanations in such a situation: chance occurrence, common genetic susceptibility and common exposure to harmful environmental (dietary) factors.

In this example the risk of large bowel cancer for first-degree relatives is derived from empirical data. Apparently, the risk is mainly dependent on the number of affected relatives and their ages at diagnosis (St John et al. 1993; Fuchs et al. 1994, Hall et al. 1994b). Various forms of surveillance have been recommended for at-risk relatives (Gaglia et al. 1995; Winawer et al. 1997).

Recent DNA studies have shed new light on the significance of young age at diagnosis of large bowel cancer. Liu et al. (1995) studied the hMSH2 and hMLH1 genes in a series of young patients with the disease. Eighteen of 31 patients (58%) who were 35 years or younger at diagnosis of colorectal cancer had MSI-positive tumours. In contrast, only 12% of tumours from patients older than 35 years were MSI-positive. Among 12 young colorectal cancer patients with a MSI-positive tumour who could be evaluated for germline mutations, five were carriers of a mutation of either the hMSH2 or hMLH1 gene. In four out of these five cases one of the parents was an asymptomatic gene carrier. The fifth parent had had large bowel cancer.

Thus, a substantial number of young patients with colorectal cancer and a negative family history may still harbour a mutation of a mismatch repair gene. It should be realized, however, that in these cases the cancer risk associated with the gene defect has not been determined. HNPCC kindreds are generally identified on the basis of a high incidence of large bowel cancer in successive generations. If in such a family a mismatch repair gene mutation is detected, this mutation is presumed to have led to the high cancer incidence. In contrast, if such a mutation is found in a sporadic patient the cancer risk associated with this gene defect may be lower than in HNPCC families. As stated by Schatzkin et al. (1995), "The excess risk of malignancy among carriers of mutant genes who are not members of cancer-prone families is unknown."

Clinical Practice: Case Histories

The following three families illustrate some of the issues discussed in the previous sections.

Case A

Kindred NL-13 (Fig. 1) demonstrates the clinical variability of HNPCC. The ages at diagnosis of colorectal cancer range from 38 to 67 years. This family includes an unaffected gene carrier (pedigree number II-1) who appears to be a case of nonpenetrance. Interestingly, the identical twin brother of the index case (pedigree numbers III-6 and III-5, respectively) has not had a colonic neoplasm. He has had a skin tumour which was either a planocellular cancer or a keratoacanthoma. One family member (pedigree number II-7) has survived multiple colonic cancers as well as ovarian and gastric cancer.

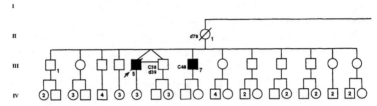

Fig. 1. Pedigree of kindred A. C, Colorectal cancer; Cx, cervical cancer; O, ovarian cancer; S, gastric (stomach) cancer; C38, age at diagnosis of colorectal cancer 38 years; d39, age at death 39 years

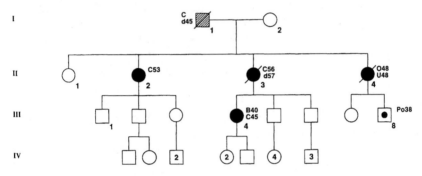

Fig. 2. Pedigree of kindred B. U, Uterine (endometrial) cancer; Po, colorectal polyp

Cervical cancer, as observed in patient III-37, is presumably unrelated to HNPCC. The condition in this kindred is due to an inactivating mutation of the hMSH2 gene. Denaturing gradient gel electrophoresis (DGGE) revealed an alteration in the hMSH2 gene, and subsequent DNA sequencing yielded the nature and site of the defect in this gene. The mutation in this kindred is a base insertion in codon 532 of exon 10 leading to termination of the translation of the gene three codons downstream (Wijnen et al. 1995). The mutation was detected in all of the investigated patients, pedigree numbers II-5, II-7, II-8, III-5, III-7 and III-37. This information offered the possibility of presymptomatic DNA-based diagnosis for high-risk family members. However, the psychosocial sequelae of DNA testing are manifold and complex. Therefore, presymptomatic DNA testing is generally conducted in three phases: pre-test counselling, the actual blood test and post-test counselling. The experience gained during the investigation and counselling of kindred NL-13 is reported elsewhere (Menko et al. 1996).

Case B

The patient discussed in this example (Fig. 2, pedigree number III-8) underwent colonoscopy at the age of 38 years. He had not been examined previously, since HNPCC had only recently been diagnosed in his family. A ses-

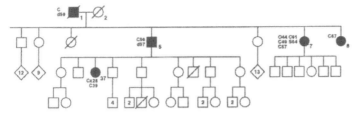

Fig. 1 (continued)

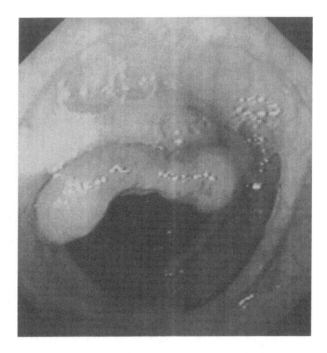

Fig. 3. Appearance at endoscopy of a sessile polyp in the transverse colon of a 38-year-old male at risk of hereditary non-polyposis colorectal cancer (Fig. 2, kindred B individual III–8). Histological examination revealed a tubulovillous adenoma with moderate dysplasia

sile polyp in the transverse colon (Fig. 3) was detected and removed endoscopically. Histological examination revealed it to be a tubulovillous adenoma with moderate dysplasia.

The mother of this patient, pedigree number II–4, was investigated at the age of 48 years due to pain in her lower abdomen. A large cystic tumour of the right ovary was biopsied and found to be malignant. Treatment consisted of hysterectomy and bilateral oophorectomy. On histological examination of the surgical specimen an endometrioid tumour of the right ovary was found and, unexpectedly, a second primary tumour (endometrioid adenocarcinoma) of the endometrium. A cousin of patient III–8, pedigree number III–4, has had both colo-

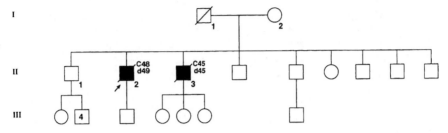

Fig. 4. Pedigree of kindred C

nic and breast cancer. We do not know whether the breast cancer is related to the HNPCC in this family. This tumour is not found more often in patients with HNPCC than in the general population (Watson and Lynch 1993).

A pathogenic mutation of the hMLH1 gene has been detected in affected family members from this kindred. This mutation was also found in family member III-8 who exhibited a tubulovillous colonic polyp at a relatively young age.

Case C

In the family depicted in Fig. 4 colorectal cancer was diagnosed in two brothers. The elder of the two patients (pedigree number II-2) had large bowel obstruction caused by sigmoidal cancer diagnosed at the age of 48 years. Since metastases were found at laparotomy, only palliative sigmoidal resection could be performed. The tumour was a moderately differentiated mucinous adenocarcinoma. Two years previously this patient's brother, pedigree number II-3, had presented at the age of 45 years with anaemia and abdominal pain. Sigmoidal cancer was diagnosed and a left hemicolectomy was performed. The surgical specimen revealed a sigmoidal adenocarcinoma, Dukes' stage C. Within a year of the diagnosis of cancer this patient died from metastatic disease. No other close relatives are affected with colorectal cancer or endometrial cancer.

In this family the cause of familial colorectal cancer has not been established. Microsatellite instability studies of the tumours from both affected relatives were negative. Periodic screening of the siblings is recommended since an increased risk of colorectal cancer is indicated by the empirical data.

Conclusions

Evaluation of the family history of patients with colorectal cancer has revealed that as many as 15% of patients report occurrence of the same disease in one or more first-degree relatives. A positive family history may have important consequences for the patient with cancer and his or her close relatives. Since management decisions should be based on a firmly established diagnosis, the family study always includes verification of the family history data by review of medical and histological reports.

The natural history of hereditary non-polyposis colorectal cancer (HNPCC) differs from that of sporadic disease. Treatment and follow-up of patients are determined by the clinical characteristics of the syndrome.

DNA-based diagnosis and presymptomatic testing will become available for an increasing number of families. For DNA testing, close cooperation between clinical and molecular geneticists is invaluable for proper evaluation of the tests. Evaluation and counselling of the family are complicated and warrant a multidisciplinary team. Teams may choose to organize a specialized cancer family clinic (Ponder 1994).

Family members at high risk of cancer may be led by fear and denial to withdraw from screening. Recognition and discussion of possible barriers to screening are therefore a critical aspect of counselling. In fact, regional or national HNPCC registries are needed to ensure surveillance of at-risk family members.

Patients with sporadic disease, especially those diagnosed at a young age, may have a genetic susceptibility to colorectal cancer.

The present state of knowledge requires that family studies, genetic counselling, DNA testing and screening be conducted in a research environment.

Acknowledgment. Figure 3 was kindly provided by the Department of Gastroenterology (head: Prof. S.G.M. Meuwissen), University Hospital Vrije Universiteit, Amsterdam

References

Aaltonen LA, Peltomäki P, Leach FS et al. (1993) Clues to the pathogenesis of familial colorectal cancer. Science 260:812–816
Fishel R, Lescoe MK, Rao MRS et al. (1993) The human mutator gene homolog MSH2 and its association with hereditary nonpolyposis colon cancer. Cell 75:1027–1038
Fuchs CS, Giovannucci EL, Colditz GA et al. (1994) A prospective study of family history and the risk of colorectal cancer. N Engl J Med 331:1669–1674
Gaglia P, Atkin WS, Whitelaw S et al. (1995) Variables associated with the risk of colorectal adenomas in asymptomatic patients with a family history of colorectal cancer. Gut 36:385–390
Hall NR, Williams MAT, Murday VA et al. (1994a) Muir-Torre syndrome: a variant of the cancer family syndrome. J Med Genet 31:627–631
Hall NR, Finan PJ, Ward B et al. (1994b) Genetic susceptibility to colorectal cancer in patients under 45 years of age. Br J Surg 81:1485–1489
Järvinen HJ, Mecklin J-P, Sistonen P (1995) Screening reduces colorectal cancer rate in families with hereditary nonpolyposis colorectal cancer. Gastroenterology 108:1405–1411
Jass JR (1995) Colorectal adenomas in surgical specimens from subjects with hereditary non-polyposis colorectal cancer. Histopathology 27:263–267
Jass JR, Stewart SM (1992) Evolution of hereditary non-polyposis colorectal cancer. Gut 33:783–786

Jass JR, Cottier DS, Jeevaratnam P et al. (1995) Diagnostic use of microsatellite instability in hereditary non-polyposis colorectal cancer. Lancet 346:1200–1201

Jass JR, Pokos V, Arnold JL et al. (1996) Colorectal neoplasms detected colonoscopically in at-risk members of colorectal cancer families stratified by the demonstration of DNA microsatellite instability. J Mol Med 74:547–551

Lanspa SJ, Jenkins JX, Cavalieri RJ et al. (1994) Surveillance in Lynch syndrome: how aggressive? Am J Gastroenterol 89:1978–1980

Leach FS, Nicolaides NC, Papadopoulos N et al. (1993) Mutations of a mutS homolog in hereditary nonpolyposis colorectal cancer. Cell 75:1215–1225

Liu B, Farrington SM, Petersen GM et al. (1995) Genetic instability occurs in the majority of young patients with colorectal cancer. Nature Med 1:348–352

Lynch HT, Smyrk TC, Watson P et al. (1993) Genetics, natural history, tumor spectrum, and pathology of hereditary nonpolyposis colorectal cancer: an updated review. Gastroenterology 104:1535–1549

Mecklin J-P, Järvinen HJ (1993) Treatment and follow-up strategies in hereditary nonpolyposis colorectal carcinoma. Dis Colon Rectum 36:927–929

Menko FH, Verheijen RHM, Vasen HFA et al. (1994) Endometrial cancer in four sisters: report of a kindred with presumed cancer family syndrome. Gynaecol Oncol 54:171–174

Menko FH, Wijnen JTh, Vasen HFA et al. (1996) Genetic counseling in hereditary nonpolyposis colorectal cancer. Oncology 10:71–76

Miyaki M, Konishi M, Tanaka K et al. (1997) Germline mutation of MSH6 as the cause of hereditary nonpolyposis colorectal cancer. Nature Genet 17:271–272

Nicolaides NC, Papadopoulos N, Liu B et al. (1994) Mutations of two PMS homologues in hereditary nonpolyposis colon cancer. Nature 371:75–80

Papadopulos N, Nicolaides NC, Wei Y-F et al. (1994) Mutation of a mutL homolog in hereditary colon cancer. Science 263:1625–1629

Ponder BAJ (1994) Setting up and running a familial cancer clinic. Br Med Bull 50:732–745

Rodríguez-Bigas MA (1996) Prophylactic colectomy for gene carriers in hereditary nonpolyposis colorectal cancer. Has the time come? Cancer 78:199–201

Schatzkin A, Goldstein A, Freedman LS (1995) What does it mean to be a cancer gene carrier? Problems in establishing causality from the molecular genetics of cancer. JNCI 87:1126–1130

Shibata D, Reale MA, Lavin P et al. (1996) The DCC protein and prognosis in colorectal cancer. N Engl J Med 335:1727–1732

StJohn DJB, McDermott FT, Hopper JL et al. (1993) Cancer risk in relatives of patients with common colorectal cancer. Ann Intern Med 118:785–790

Vasen HFA, Mecklin J-P, Meera Khan P et al. (1991) The International Collaborative Group on Hereditary Nonpolyposis Colorectal Cancer (ICG-HNPCC). Dis Colon Rectum 34:424–425

Vasen HFA, Taal BG, Griffioen G et al. (1994) Clinical heterogeneity of familial colorectal cancer and its influence on screening protocols. Gut 35:1262–1266

Vasen HFA, Nagengast FM, Meera Khan P (1995) Interval cancers in hereditary non-polyposis colorectal cancer (Lynch syndrome). Lancet 345:1183–1184

Vasen HFA, Wijnen J Th, Menko FH et al. (1996) Cancer risk in families with hereditary nonpolyposis colorectal cancer diagnosed by mutation analysis. Gastroenterology 110:1020–1027

Water van de NS, Stewart SM, Jeevaratnam P et al. (1994) Direct mutational analysis in a family with hereditary non-polyposis colorectal cancer. Aust N Z Med 24:682–686

Watson P, Lynch HT (1993) Extracolonic cancer in hereditary nonpolyposis colorectal cancer. Cancer 71:677–685

Watson P, Vasen HFA, Mecklin JP, Lynch HT (1994) The risk of endometrial cancer in hereditary nonpolyposis colorectal cancer. Am J Med 96:516–520

Winawer SJ, Fletcher RH, Miller R et al. (1997) Colorectal cancer screening: clinical guidelines and rationale. Gastroenterology 112:594–642

Wijnen J, Vasen H, Meera Khan P et al. (1995) Seven new mutations in hMSH2 (an HNPCC gene) identified by denaturing gradient-gel electrophoresis (DGGE). Am J Hum Genet 56:1060-1066

Wijnen J, Meera Khan P, Vasen H et al. (1996) Majority of hMLH1 mutations responsible for hereditary nonpolyposis colorectal cancer (HNPCC) cluster at the exonic region 15-16. Am J Hum Genet 58:300-307

Wijnen J, Meera Khan P, Vasen H et al. (1997) Hereditary nonpolyposis colorectal cancer families not complying with the Amsterdam criteria show extremely low frequency of mismatch-repair-gene mutations. Am J Hum Genet 61:329-335

Staging and Prognostic Markers

Use and Applications of MRI Techniques in the Diagnosis and Staging of Rectal Lesions

T. J. Vogl[1], W. Pegios[1], M. Hünerbein[2], M. G. Mack[1], P. M. Schlag[2] and R. Felix[1]

[1] Department of Radiology, Virchow Hospital, Humboldt University of Berlin, Augustenburger Platz 1, 13353 Berlin, Germany
[2] Department of Surgery and Surgical Oncology, Robert-Rössle-Hospital, Humboldt University of Berlin, Lindenberger Weg 80, 13122 Berlin, Germany

Introduktion

Each year, 100000–150000 new cases of colorectal carcinoma occur in the USA, with an almost equal incidence in both sexes (Whalen 1990). According to the American Cancer Society, the incidence of and mortality from colorectal cancer in the USA are second after lung cancer in men and third in women; the incidence rose by 9.4% between 1973 and 1986. Dietary factors, family history, a variety of polyposis syndromes, and long-standing inflammatory bowel disease are risk factors for the development of colorectal carcinoma.

Because specific treatment options will vary with tumor location, the preoperative evaluation of rectal carcinoma is important for therapy planning and assessment of the prognosis. So far there are several limitations on determining the width and depth of infiltration of the wall layers in rectal tumors (adenoma and carcinoma) by the usual endoscopic and X-ray procedures (barium enema, computed tomography), endosonography, and conventional magnetic resonance imaging.

Barium sulfate enema and/or flexible sigmoidoscopy are the primary examinations used in the evaluation of the rectum and sigmoid colon. Both are excellent modalities, showing the mucosal surface with exquisite detail. Sigmoidoscopy is helpful for the evaluation of macroscopic aspects, localization of the lesion, and morphology including tactile and visual characteristics. Additional advantages are the possibility of biopsy and the decision about the final treatment modality.

Staging with computed tomography (CT) is accurate in 48%–74% of cases (Moss 1989). Early studies using magnetic resonance imaging (MRI) failed to show greater accuracy than CT (Butch et al. 1986). In particular, initial studies showed that depiction of tumor infiltration on MRI through the bowel wall was difficult. Transrectal ultrasound is now an established imaging modality for evaluation of the integrity of the wall layers in the vicinity of colorectal lesions (Rifkin and Marks 1985). Overstaging seems the most frequent error, both in staging of rectal cancer (Tio et al. 1991) and screening of adenomas for invasive malignancy (Hulsmans et al. 1992).

MRI imaging is helpful for tumor staging and the detection of tumor recurrence, and especially aids in clarifying questions remaining after endoscopic diagnosis. Patient movement must be minimized in order to improve image quality. The use of rapid scanning techniques, endoluminal surface coils, and paramagnetic contrast agents especially is expanding the applications of MRI in the evaluation of rectal and perirectal disease. Specimen studies using surface coils and preliminary clinical studies using endorectal coils have shown great promise for the assessment of local tumor extent (Chan et al. 1991; Schnall et al. 1994; Pegios et al. 1996a).

Recommended MRI Sequences

Whenever possible, rectum and sigmoid should be cleansed with enemas before MRI, as sometimes retained fecal material cannot be differentiated from tumor. When using an endorectal surface coil, digital examination of the rectum should be performed before placement to ensure there are no obstructions within the lumen. The distance from the rectal lesion to the anus should be determined before hand during barium enema study and sigmoidoscopy. The center of the endorectal coil is positioned at the center of the lesion. To minimize motion artifacts produced by bowel contractions, glucacon or similar antiperistaltic medications are recommended. The position of the endorectal coil is checked with a sagittal localizer with the patient supine.

Whatever the field strength, T1- and T2-weighted spin-echo sequences are recommended as the basic technique when using the body coil. T1-w images provide an excellent outline of the bowel wall, show intraluminal masses, and demonstrate changes affecting the extravesical fat. T2-w images show tissue changes in the bowel wall (neoplastic or inflammatory), as well as better characterization of extracolonic masses. For comparative evaluation an additional turbo SE sequence is performed. At the slice position where the tumor appears largest, dynamic endorectal MRI may be performed starting with a bolus of 0.1 mmol/kg b.w. Gd-DTPA (Schering, Berlin, Germany) in order to evaluate the dynamic contrast enhancement. Axial and sagittal T1-w sequences are then performed (Tables 1, 2). Imaging in the sagittal plane provides information on the anterior and posterior relationships of the rectum and sigmoid colon.

MRI Appearance

Normal Findings

The zonal anatomy of the rectal wall is best appreciated in transverse-plane images. The perirectal space is also easily assessed in the transverse plane. Plain MRI using the *body coil* demonstrates a high soft-tissue contrast of ad-

Table 1. MRI protocol 1: plain imaging

Coil	Sequence	TR/TE	FOV	Sd	Matrix	Plane
Body	T2 SE	2500/22-90	350	4	256×512	Transverse
Endorectal	T2 SE	2500/22-90	160	4	160×512	Transverse
	Turbo TSE	3700/90	160	4	192×256	Transverse
	T1 SE	700/15	1180	4	180×512	Transverse

Table 2. MRI protocol 2: dynamic imaging with Gd-DTPA[a]

Coil	Sequence	TR/TE	FOV	Sd	Matrix	Plane
Endorectal turbo	FLASH	7/3	160	1	128×128	Transverse
	T1 SE	700/15	180	4	180×512	Transverse
	T1 SE	700/15	180	4	180×512	Sagittal

[a] 0.1 mmol/kg body weight.

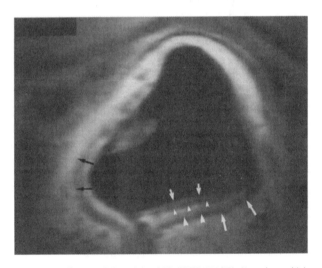

Fig. 1. Endorectal MRI of the normal rectal wall (sagittal T1-weighted SE, TR/TE=700/15). Note the multiple layers visualized in the rectal wall: high-signal-intensity mucus within the rectal lumen (*short white arrows*), low-signal-intensity mucosal layer (mucosa and muscularis mucosa) (*small white arrowheads*), high-signal-intensity submucosal layer (*large white arrowheads*), low-signal-intensity muscularis propria (*long white arrows*), and high-signal-intensity perirectal fat (*black arrows*)

jacent structures and allows the mucosa to be made out as a band of high signal intensity in the T2-w sequence, surrounded by a layer of low signal intensity relating to the muscularis propria. If the rectum is imaged following intravenous administration of Gd-DTPA, the enhancement of submucosa and mucosa allows the layers of rectal wall to be distinguished on T1-w scans. Further visual identification of other rectal layers is uncertain.

Table 3. TNM staging for cancer of the colon and rectum

Stage	Level of involvement
Tumor	
Tx	Tumor cannot be assessed
T0	No evidence of tumor
Tis	Carcinoma in situ[a]
T1	Tumor invades the submucosa
T2	Tumor invades the muscularis propria
T3	Tumor invades through the muscularis propria into the subserosa or into nonperitonealized pericolic or perirectal tissues
T4	Tumor invades other organs or structures
Nodes	
Nx	Regional lymph nodes cannot be assessed
N0	No involved lymph nodes
N1	Fewer than four regional nodes positive for tumor
N2	More than four regional nodes positive for tumor
N3	Central nodes positive for tumor

From: American Joint Committee on Cancer (1992) Manual for staging of cancer, 4th edn. Lippincott, Philadelphia
[a] Cancer cells within basement membrane or lamina propria with no extension through the muscularis propria into the submucosa.

Plain and contrast-enhanced MRI with the *endorectal surface coil* using T2-w and T1-w sequences allows identification of all the layers of the circumference of the rectal wall (Fig. 1). These layers consist of an inner layer of medium signal intensity (the mucus and fluid between the coil and the rectal wall), a layer of low signal intensity (mucosa and muscularis mucosa), a middle layer of medium-to-high signal intensity (the submucosa), a second layer of low signal intensity (the muscularis propria), and an outer layer of high signal intensity (the perirectal fat) in the T1-w sequence. On T2-w spin-echo images the inner layer (mucus and fluid between the coil and the rectal wall) and the middle layer (the submucosa) are shown with a high signal intensity.

Pathologic Findings

MRI staging of colorectal cancer can follow the suggested TNM classification (Table 3). MRI is not applicable to the assessment of stage Tis.

Using conventional MRI rectal carcinomas are demonstrated at a high signal intensity in the T2-w sequence and are thus more conspicuous than in T1-w images. Infiltration of the bowel wall is best demonstrated in T2-w scans, because these images best show normal zonal anatomy of the wall and because the contrast between the high signal intensity of tumors and low signal intensity of muscle tissue is maximized. Perirectal fat and soft-tissue in-

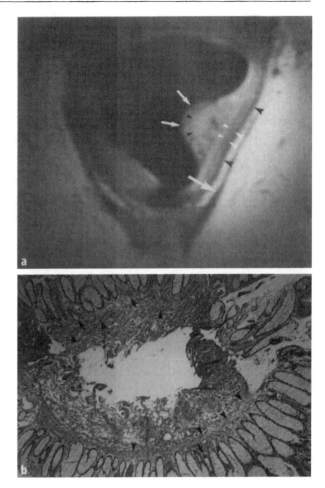

Fig. 2. a Endorectal MRI (T1-weighted SE, 700/15, after administration of 0.1 mmol/kg b.w. Gd-DTPA) demonstrates a small pedunculate adenoma of the rectum. The different layers of the rectal wall can be identified. From lateral to medial: high signal intensity of the perirectal fat tissue, followed by the low signal intensity of the muscularis propria (*large black arrowheads*), followed by a layer of high signal intensity representing the submucosal core (*large white arrowheads*), low signal intensity of the muscularis mucosa (*small white arrowheads*), and the low signal intensity of the thickened mucosal layer (*small black arrowheads*) with mucus within the rectal lumen (*small white arrows*). The (*large white arrow*) indicates the levator ani muscle.
b Histologic section demonstrates the normal muscularis mucosa (*arrowheads*) and the thickened mucosa with typical grade II–III dysplasia (*arrows*)

filtration by tumor will be most conspicuous in T1-w images. Rectal carcinomas enhance following administration of Gd-DTPA, and Gd-DTPA-enhanced T1-w images help in determining the depth of tumor growth.

Endorectal MRI enables correct identification of all layers of the rectal wall and differentiation between the different tumor stages.

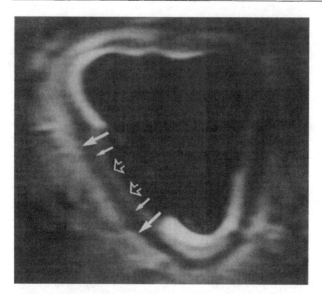

Fig. 3. Eight weeks after electrolaser resection of a tubulovillous adenoma. The endorectal surface coil image again gives a clear visualization of the different rectal layers. This turbo spin-echo image (TR/TE=3700/90) shows a slight increase of signal intensity and edematous infiltration of the remaining parts of the submucosa (*open white arrows*). *Short white arrows*; muscularis propria; *long white arrows*, perirectal fat

Rectal Adenoma

The following have been defined as general criteria for diagnosis of an adenoma: visualization of an intact muscularis mucosa, clear demarcation of the submucosa, sharp borders of the lesion, and high homogeneous contrast enhancement of the lesion in dynamic turbo FLASH sequences. In T2-w sequences the tumors characteristically show as a homogeneous high signal intensity, brighter than the surrounding structures. Plain T1-w sequences are best for exact delineation of the lesions against the different wall layers (Fig. 2). Contrast-enhanced T1-w sequences reveal nearly homogeneous contrast enhancement of the tumor. In all tumors we observed significantly higher contrast enhancement of the mucosal layer than of the tumor tissue.

Follow-up studies of patients with large tubulovillous adenomas demonstrate total removal of the tumor after endoscopic electrolaser resection (Fig. 3). After treatment, MRI with the endorectal surface coil demonstrates resection of the mucosa and parts of the submucosa. Again, clear visualization of the different rectal layers is possible. Only T2-w and turbo spin-echo images showed a slight increase in signal intensity and edematous infiltration of the submucosa at the former location of the adenoma due to ongoing repair activity.

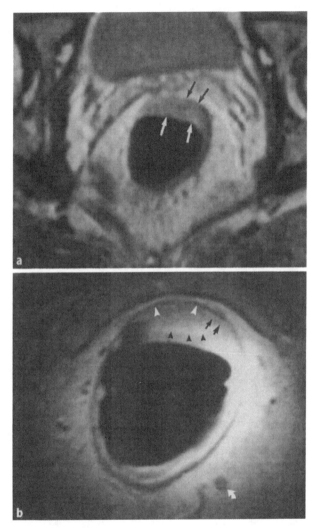

Fig. 4. a Conventional axial T2-weighted SE image (TR/TE=2500/22) demonstrates a sessile lesion of the ventral circumference of the rectum (*white arrows*) with suspected extension into the muscularis propria (*black arrows*); this was initially mistakenly staged as T2 cancer. **b** Endorectal MRI (T2-weighted SE, TR/TE=2500/22) reveals the lesion as focal mucosal thickening (*black arrowheads*) with a high-signal-intensity submucosal core (*black arrows*); the muscularis propria (*white arrowheads*) has not been involved. Additionally, one small, 3-mm-diameter perirectal lymph node has been completely replaced by soft tissue (*curved white arrow*). This was positive for carcinoma at pathologic examination. (Final staging was pT1N1)

Rectal Carcinoma

The presence of mucosal thickening with preservation of the submucosal layer is indicative of a stage T1 lesion. A possible error in endorectal MRI is overestimation of T1 lesions as T2 lesions. This is caused by thinning of the

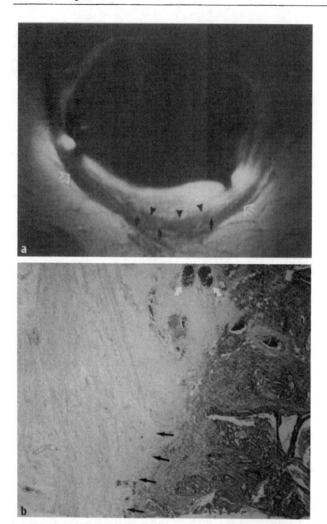

Fig. 5. a Endorectal MRI imaging (T1-weighted SE, TR/TE=700/15) after administration of contrast medium (0.1 mmol/kg b.w. Gd-DTPA) visualizes a clearly demarcated lesion (*black arrowheads*) with increased contrast enhancement and a suspected irregular extension into the muscularis propria (*black arrows*). *open arrow*, Levator ani muscle. **b** Histopathologic study (hematoxylin-eosin) reveals incipient infiltration into but not through the muscularis propria (*straight arrows*). *Curved arrows*, Vessels

muscularis propria with compression and nonvisualization of the submucosa (mechanical compression) near the base of the lesion (Fig. 4). The dynamic turbo FLASH sequence is helpful in distinguishing an intact muscularis propria without suspicious irregularities.

The defined MRI criteria for a stage T2 carcinoma – extension of the tumor into but not through the muscularis propria – are a mass of high signal intensity in the T2-w images with in a band of low signal intensity. The partially intact muscularis propria does not show significant contrast enhance-

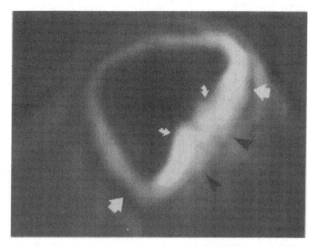

Fig. 6. Dynamic turbo FLASH sequence (TR/TE/TI=7/3/300, flip angle = 15°) after administration of contrast medium (0.1 mmol/kg b.w. Gd-DTPA) obtained in a patient with a sessile rectal lesion reveals, inhomogeneous contrast enhancement of the lesion (*curved white arrows*) and complete disruption of the muscularis propria with a blurred border with the perirectal fat tissue (*black arrowheads*). *Wide white arrows,* Muscularis propria

ment in T1-w sequences. The tumor tissue, however, displays high contrast enhancement, thus serving as a valid criterion for diagnosing a stage T2 lesion. Sometimes the irregularity of the border between the muscularis propria and the perirectal fat tissue in the T1-w sequence makes staging difficult and leads to an overestimation as a T3 tumor. However, the dynamic turbo FLASH sequence and turbo spin-echo T2-w sequence show clear demarcation of the muscularis propria without infiltration of the perirectal fat tissue (Fig. 5).

Both conventional and endorectal MRI are useful in identifying stage T3 and T4 disease. Complete disruption of the muscularis propria and a blurred border with the perirectal fat tissue are the criteria for a T3 lesion (Fig. 6). A T4 lesion shows infiltration of adjacent structures.

On the T1-w images, the rectal wall gives a relatively homogeneous intermediate signal intensity pattern. These images provide good contrast between the perirectal fat and the bowel wall and are helpful for identifying perirectal vessels and lymph nodes. Both conventional and endorectal MRI can also be used for lymph node evaluation. Pararectal nodes 1 cm or greater in size can be detected in multiple planes with conventional MRI, while high-resolution endorectal MRI is excellent for depicting perirectal nodes as small as 5 mm in diameter (Fig. 4b). Inflammatory nodes cannot be differentiated from metastatic nodes on the basis of size or signal intensity.

Discussion

Accurate preoperative staging has a definite impact on the surgical management of rectal carcinoma. The standard surgical treatment for rectal cancer is abdominoperineal resection (Curley et al. 1989). However, because of the morbidity associated with this procedure, the most notable of which are the social and physical problems of a permanent colostomy, a number of alternative surgical approaches have been proposed. These include anus-sparing radical resections such as low anterior resection (Rothenberger and Wong 1985) and local excision (Hager et al. 1983), and nonsurgical approaches such as low-kilovoltage endorectal irradiation electrocautery, and transanal fulguration. Consequently, accurate staging of the local extent of rectal cancer is important to the successful enforcement of any conservative treatment regimen. In addition, the preoperative staging is important in selecting patients for planned adjuvant preoperative radiation therapy, chemotherapy, and hyperthermia therapy.

Radiological modalities that have been used in the staging of rectal carcinoma include computed tomography (CT), transrectal ultrasonography, and MRI. The accuracy of staging with CT was reported to be as high as 90% in initial reports (Thoeni et al. 1981). Later published articles showed that CT studies are of limited usefulness for accurate staging of local disease or depth of wall invasion (Hodgman et al. 1986). CT does not permit evaluation of less extensive tumors because differentiation of the normal layers of the intestinal wall is impossible due to the poor soft tissue contrast. A recent study showed the sensitivity and specificity of CT for the detection of extension of perirectal fat to be lower than those of MRI and endorectal ultrasound (Rifkin et al. 1989). Tumors located low in the rectum were particularly difficult to stage because of the paucity of perirectal fat in this region (Hodgman et al. 1986).

Transrectal ultrasonography is now an established imaging modality for evaluation of the integrity of the wall layers underneath the colorectal lesion (Rifkin and Marks 1985). Some authors have reported it to be 77% accurate in demonstrating invasion of carcinoma into the perirectal fat and 50% accurate in demonstrating perirectal lymph node involvement (Rifkin et al. 1989). New articles report 75%–83% accuracy for staging rectal cancer with transrectal ultrasonography (Milsom and Graffner 1990). However, this imaging modality does not provide reliable contrast between the tumor and the muscularis propria. Thus, once the submucosa is breached, it is often difficult to determine the depth of muscle invasion and to detect early perirectal fat invasion. In addition, the ability of different ultrasound characteristics to differentiate between T2 and T3 tumors is limited. Spontaneous or iatrogenic inflammation is a major limiting factor (Hulsmans et al. 1994). Often in follow-up examinations with transrectal sonography the inflammatory changes in the rectal wall after treatment of colorectal adenoma with photocoagulation may simulate malignant infiltration (during about the first 6 weeks) (Hulsmans et al. 1993).

Complete removal of adenomatous polyps is the most important measure in prophylaxis of colorectal adenocarcinomas (Shinya and Wolff 1979). Laser photocoagulation is often used for sessile villous adenomas in patients with a poor surgical or medical condition (Mathus-Vliegen and Tytgat 1986).

Few articles have been published about the use of MRI with a body coil to stage rectal carcinoma (Butch et al. 1986; Hodgman et al. 1986). The depth of bowel wall invasion cannot be determined, and the accuracy of staging with conventional MRI has been reported as no higher than 60% (Hodgman et al 1986). The limitation of conventional MRI in initial studies was inadequate resolution. De Lange et al. (1990) described results with an external surface coil for MRI of rectal cancer. They were able to decrease voxel volume to 5.7 mm^3 and reported a high accuracy in identifying lesions invading perirectal fat (89%). The usefulness of this technique in reduced in obese patients because the sensitive volume of the surface coil configuration is limited to approximately one radius.

Several authors have reported on the use of a high-resolution endorectal surface coil. They have reported an accuracy of 81%–85% in staging the extent of the primary lesion in rectal carcinoma, which is better than reported for CT and body coil MRI and similar to that claimed for endorectal ultrasonography (Chan et al. 1991; Schnall et al. 1994; Pegios et al. 1996a). The layers of the rectal wall were visible in all cases. An important point is that none of the cases were understaged: this prevents patients with highly invasive disease from being undertreated. In addition, these authors reported a specifity of 72% for N1 disease in demonstrating perirectal adenopathy (Schnall et al 1994).

Follow-up studies have shown that endorectal surface coil MRI is probably better than transrectal ultrasonography for assessing patients after electrolaser resection (Pegios et al. 1996b), because it is so easy to misinterpret inflammatory changes using transrectal ultrasonography.

Nevertheless, some problems still remain in using the endorectal surface coil. Presumably because the pressure of the balloon presses the low-signal-intensity mucosa and muscularis propria together, it is difficult to identify the layers. Another limitation in the staging of rectal neoplasms by endorectal MRI is benign peritumoral inflammatory reaction spreading into the outer muscular layer, making it difficult to differentiate between T2 and T3 rectal cancer.

Although high-resolution endorectal MRI is excellent for depicting perirectal nodes larger than 3 mm in diameter, inflammatory nodes cannot be differentiated from metastatic nodes in regard to size or signal intensity pattern (Schnall et al. 1994; Pegios et al. 1996). Further studies are needed to assess the architecture, geometry, and contrast enhancement characteristics of lymph nodes.

Turbo spin-echo images are useful for reliable depiction of the bowel wall architecture. The dynamic turbo FLASH sequence is helpful in the differentiation between tumor stage T2 and T3 (Pegios et al. 1996), because it more reliably shows any muscularis propria involvement or complete disrupture of the muscularis propria.

Additional studies are necessary to further establish criteria for interpreting high-resolution rectal images, and intraindividual comparisons of endorectal MRI versus endorectal ultrasonography are also needed.

References

Butch RJ, Stark DD, Wittenberg J (1986) Staging rectal cancery by MR and CT. AJR 146:1155-1160

Chan TW, Kressel HY, Milestone B et al. (1991) Rectal carcinoma: staging at MR imaging with endorectal surface coil-work in progress. Radiology 181:461-467

Curley SA, Roh MS, Rich TA (1989) Surgical therapy of early rectal carcinoma. Hematol Oncol Clin North Am 3:87-101

de Lange EE, Fechner RE, Edge SB, Spaulding CA (1990) Preoperative staging of rectal carcinoma with MR imaging: surgical and histopathologic correlation. Radiology 176:623-628

Hager TH, Gall FP, Hermanek P (1983) Local excision of cancer of the rectum. Dis Colon Rectum 26:149-151

Hodgman CG, MacCarty RL, Wolf BG et al. (1986) Preoperative staging of rectal carcinoma by computed tomography and 0.15T magnetic resonance imaging. Colon Rectum 29:446-450

Hulsmans FJH, Tio TL, Mathus-Vliegen EMH, Bosma A, Tytgat GNJ (1992) Colorectal villous adenoma: transrectal US in screening for invasive malignancy. Radiology 185:193-196

Hulsmans FJH, Mathus-Vliegen, Bosman S, Bosma A, Tytgat GNJ (1993) Colorectal adenomas: inflammatory changes that simulate malignancy after laser coagulation-evaluation with transrectal US. Radiology 187:367-371

Hulsmans FJH, Tio TL, Fockens P, Bosma A, Tytgat GNJ (1994) Assessment of tumor infiltration depth in rectal cancer with transrectal sonography: caution is necessary. Radiology 190:715-720

Mathus-Vliegen EMH, Tytgat GNJ (1986) Nd:YAG laser photocoagulation in colorectal adenomas: evaluation of its safety, usefulness and efficacy. Gastroenterology 90:1865-1873

Milsom JW, Graffner H (1990) Intrarectal ultrasonography in rectal cancer staging and in the evaluation of pelvic disease: clinical uses of intrarectal ultrasound. Ann Surg 212:602-606

Moss AA (1989) Imaging of colorectal carcinoma. Radiology 170:308-310

Pegios W, Vogl THJ, Mack MG, Hünerbein M et al. (1996b) MRI diagnosis and staging of rectal carcinoma. Abdom Imaging 21 (3)

Pegios W, Vogl TJ, Hünerbein M, Mack MG et al. (1996a) Hochauflösende Magnetresonanztomographie mittels Endorektalspule. Ergebnisse bei Tumoren des Rektums. Fortschr Röntgenstr (RÖFO) 5:17-23

Rifkin MD, Marks GJ (1985) Transrectal US as an adjunct in the diagnosis of rectal and extrarectal tumors. Radiology 157:499-502

Rifkin MD, Ehrlich SM, Marks G (1989) Staging of rectal carcinoma: prospective comparison of endorectal US and CT. Radiology 170:319-322

Rothenberger DA, Wong WD (1985) Rectal cancer: adequacy of surgical management. Ann Surg 17:309-312

Schnall MD, Furth EE, Rosato EF, Kressel HY (1994) Rectal tumor stage: Correlation of endorectal MR imaging and pathologic findings. Radiology 190:709-714

Shinya H, Wolff W (1979) Morphology, anatomic distribution and cancer potential of colonic polyps: an analysis of 7000 polyps endoscopically removed. Ann Surg 190:679-683

Thoeni R, Moss AA, Schnyder P, Margulis AR (1981) Detection and staging of primary rectal and rectosigmoid cancer by computed tomography. Radiology 141:135-138

Tio TL, Coene PPLO, van Delden OM, Tytgat GNJ (1991) Colorectal carcinoma: preoperative TNM classification with endosonography. Radiology 179:165–170

Whalen E (1990) Colon cancer: diagnosis in an era of cost containment. CR conference, November 8, 1989. AJR 154:875–881

The Value of Tumor Markers in Colorectal Cancer

M. Hünerbein

Department of Surgery and Surgical Oncology, Robert Rössle Hospital, Humboldt University of Berlin, Lindenberger Weg 80, 13122 Berlin, Germany

Abstract

Currently CEA is the most accurate tumor marker for colorectal cancer. Preoperative determination of this marker can assist staging, treatment planning and in particular postoperative follow-up of colorectal cancer. Postoperative CEA monitoring should be performed every 3 months. Further evaluation for local recurrence or metastatic disease is mandatory if elevated or increasing CEA levels occur after radical surgery. However, present data do not justify using CEA alone for postoperative follow-up and monitoring of adjuvant therapy. Molecular genetic techniques are now increasingly performed to detect genetic alterations that can be used as prognostic markers. In the future, identification and quantification of these genes may even be valuable in defining the susceptibility of healthy individuals for colorectal cancer.

Introduction

In the western world adenocarcinomas of the colon and rectum affect approximately one person in 20 and represent 15% of all cancers in the United States (Cohen 1996). Recently, on the basis of data from the Connecticut Tumor Registry, it has been shown that the incidence of colorectal cancer has been increasing over the last 50 years (Vukasin et al. 1990). The age-adjusted incidence of colon cancer increased at a constant rate, whereas the incidence of rectal cancer remained unchanged.

These data demonstrate that colorectal cancer constitutes a major health problem in western countries. Consequently considerable efforts have been made to elucidate the risk factors, etiology and biological behavior of colorectal cancer and to understand the significance of these factors for stage-adjusted treatment. Some success has now been achieved, with a 10% increase in the 5-year survival rate compared to 1950 (Cohen 1996).

In the last 20 years tumor markers for colorectal cancer have been evaluated extensively because it was hoped that therapeutic decisions could be guided by these markers, thus improving the outcome of the patients. Tumor markers are defined as biomolecules that are produced preferentially by tumor cells and can indicate the presence, extent and future behavior of cancer. The reasons for determining tumor markers are to detect tumors at an early stage, diagnose metastatic disease, and predict the prognosis. In addition, tumor markers can be useful in diagnosing recurrent disease and monitoring the success of treatment. More recently, molecular genetic techniques have been used as prognostic indicators and to identify risk groups with a genetic predisposition for the development of cancer.

Screening

Screening for colorectal cancer is a diagnostic concept that is applied to asymptomatic patients for the early detection of premalignant lesions or cancer. Because colorectal cancer is frequently preceded by precursor lesions such as adenoma, the goal of most screening programs is to detect such lesions. Testing for fecal occult blood is one of the most common screening procedures for colorectal tumors. A large trial involving more than 45 000 persons has demonstrated that the mortality from colorectal cancer can be reduced by 33% if fecal blood tests are performed (Mandel et al. 1993). However, a major problem with this method is the high rate of false positive results (approximately 30%–50%), which are followed by unnecessary colonoscopy (Cummings et al. 1986; Morris et al. 1991). Endoscopy can cause considerable discomfort for patients and may be associated with a complication rate of 1/2000–3000. Additionally, using colonoscopy to screen for large bowel cancer seems unjustifiable because of its high cost to the community.

The value of serum carcinoembryonic antigen (CEA) in screening for colorectal cancer has been investigated in multiple studies. The detection rate for colon cancer ranged from 0.1% to 4%, which means that 250 false positive results must be accepted for the detection of one person with cancer (Costanza et al. 1974; Fletcher 1986; Stevens et al. 1975).

In the last few years molecular genetic techniques have been increasingly employed to elucidate the molecular basis of malignant cell transformation and to identify patients at high risk of cancer. Overexpression of c-*myc* and k-*ras* oncogenes may play an important role in the development of colorectal cancer (Benhattar et al. 1993). In the future identification and quantification of these genes may be valuable in defining the susceptibility of healthy individuals to developing colorectal cancer. One of the first approaches to utilizing genetic alterations for screening for colorectal cancer was to examine feces for cells with k-*ras* mutations (Sidransky et al. 1992). Mutations of the k-*ras* oncogene are found in approximately 40% of colorectal carcinomas. Using a modified PCR technique, Wagner (1996) was able to identify k-*ras* mutations in 15 of 18 patients (83%) with k-*ras*-positive tumors.

It has been recognized that two forms of familial colorectal cancer exist, referred to respectively as familial adenomatous polyposis (FAP) and hereditary nonpolyposis colorectal cancer (HNPCC). Because both are inherited in a mendelian pattern, genetic evaluation of individuals with a family history could be valuable in reducing the incidence of colorectal cancer and it associated mortality.

The more important heritable syndrome is FAP, because it follows an autosomal dominant pattern with 90% penetrance. Without intervention virtually all affected persons develop colorectal cancer. To date the syndrome has been diagnosed on the basis of family history and clinical features, in particular the occurrence of more than 100 colonic polyps. The affected gene, referred to as the APC gene, has been identified on the long arm of chromosome 5 (5q21:APC) (Bodmer et al. 1987). Genetic markers are now available that can be used for the recognition of individuals who possess the inherited gene but have not yet developed the phenotypic manifestations. Surgical treatment can be offered to these individuals, thus preventing the hazardous sequelae of the genetic defect. On the other hand unnecessary screening procedures such as colonoscopy may be avoided in relatives who do not carry the gene – and at the same time the latter can be reassured that their risk is no higher than that of the general population.

HNPCC, also refered to as Lynch syndrome, is a disease characterized by the occurrence of cancer in patients younger than 50 years (Boland and Troncale 1984). The diagnosis of HNPCC is based on the Amsterdam criteria. Experimental investigations are currently underway to determine the genetic alterations that are associated with the disease. Microsatellite instability has been found in almost all persons with HNPCC and 12%–15% of sporadic cases. Furthermore, at least four HNPCC genes have been described – hMSH2, hMLH1, hPMS1, and hPMS2 – in germline cells of families with HNPCC (Altonen and Peltomaki 1994; Fishel et al. 1994; Lynch et al. 1993). However, genetic markers suitable for routine clinical evaluation of families with HNPCC are not yet available.

Pretherapeutic Assessment of Prognosis

Pretherapeutic assessment of the prognosis is of major importance for therapeutic strategy in patients with colorectal cancer. Various concepts are available for stage-adjusted therapy of colorectal cancer, including extensive resections, sphincter-preserving procedures, and combined modality therapy. There is evidence that preoperative radiotherapy has the potential to reduce the risk of local recurrence and to improve the resectability of advanced rectal cancer (Baigrie and Berry 1994). Furthermore, it has been shown that preoperative radiochemotherapy can improve the survival rate. However, the selection criteria for patients who will benefit from neoadjuvant therapy remain unclear. On the other hand, appropriate markers could avoid unnecessary treatment in patients with a low probability of recurrence or metastatic disease.

The prognostic value of CEA determinations in patients with colorectal cancer has been studied extensively. Wolmark et al. (1984) found highly significant differences in the CEA levels between patients with different Dukes stage tumors: the mean CEA value was 4 ng/ml for Dukes stage A tumors compared to 32 ng/ml for Dukes stage C tumors. Several authors have reported, that the risk of postoperative recurrence increases with increasing CEA levels. Steele et al. (1982) observed recurrent disease in 31% of the patients with Dukes stage B2 or C tumors and CEA levels of more than 5 ng/ml, but only in only 18% of the patients with CEA levels of less than 5 ng/ml ($p = 0.03$).

Others have correlated preoperative CEA levels with the survival of the patients. In a study involving more than 100 patients, CEA levels of less than 30 ng/ml were associated with a better 5-year survival rate than higher values (Laurent-Puig et al. 1992). In a large trial, approximately 1800 patients were divided into three groups with normal (1-7 ng/ml), elevated (8-15 ng/ml), or markedly elevated (>15 ng/ml) preoperative CEA levels (Sener et al. 1989). The 5-year survival rates were 61%, 50%, and 32% respectively for patients with Dukes stage B2/3 tumors and 44%, 30%, and 26% respectively for patients with Dukes stage C2/3 tumors ($p<0.0058$).

Understanding the molecular genetic mechanisms that induce progression from adenoma to carcinoma may be the key to improved detection of risk groups. Various genetic alterations have been found in colon tumors, including mutations in chromosome 5, the *ras* gene (chromosome 12), mutation and deletion of the *p53* gene (chromosome 17p), and deleted colon cancer gene (chromosome 18q) (Jen et al. 1994; Kern et al. 1992; Kinzler et al. 1991; Vogelstein et al. 1988).

During the last few years the search for micrometastases has been introduced as a potential tool for identification of patients at high risk of metastatic disease. Immunocytochemistry is most commonly used for the detection of micrometastases of solid tumors in the blood or the bone marrow. With this technique, staining of single tumor cells is carried out using monoclonal antibodies directed against tissue-specific gene products. Antibodies against the epithelial marker CK18 or CEA have been favored for colorectal cancer. One disadvantage of this method is that the sensitivity depends on the number of cells investigated and the experience of the pathologist. Recent data suggest that nested PCR can improve detection of metastatic tumor cells (Gerhard et al. 1994). Neumaier et al. (1995) were able to detect single CEA-expressing tumor cells reliably among 2×10^7 normal bone marrow cells. On the other hand, amplification of CEA mRNA was never observed in bone marrow samples from healthy donors. It would appear that in the future molecular genetic techniques will improve risk assessment, thus allowing a better stage-adjusted approach to therapy.

Detection of Tumor Recurrence

Despite apparently radical resection, 20%-30% of patients with rectal cancer develop local recurrence (Stipa et al. 1991). Furthermore, metachronous liver metastases will be diagnosed in 30%–50% of patients after resection of colorectal primaries. Complete resection remains the most effective treatment for local recurrence or liver metastases of colorectal cancer. It has been shown that resection of up to three liver metastases improves the survival of patients significantly (Schlag et al. 1996). Therefore follow-up programs after surgery for rectal cancer aim at the detection of recurrence at early and potentially curable stages.

According to the guidelines of the American Society of Clinical Oncology, only CEA has proved its major role in the postoperative follow-up of colorectal cancer (ASCO 1996). Residual disease is likely if CEA concentrations remain elevated more than 6 weeks postoperatively. However 10%–20% of colorectal carcinomas are not accompanied by elevation of tumor markers despite distant metastases, while on the other hand cross-reacting antigens as well as nicotine abuse, bronchitis, liver cirrhosis, and chronic inflammatory bowel disease can lead to false positive findings.

Generally, increasing serum CEA after curative resection of colorectal cancer can indicate tumor recurrence, even if the absolute value remains within the normal range. In addition to the absolute serum concentrations, the doubling time of CEA levels is a useful parameter for the assessment of tumor burden. It has been shown that distant metastases induce a faster increase per month (10%) than local recurrence (5%) (Steele et al. 1982). There is also some evidence that tumor marker determinations may be more sensitive than imaging studies. In a study by Ward et al. (1993) tumor marker pattern suggested recurrence 4 months before the lesion was detected by imaging methods. However, it has not yet been established that chemotherapy because of elevated CEA values alone can improve survival. Therefore second-look laparotomy should be considered in selected patients with rising CEA levels to avoid further progression of occult recurrences. It has been reported that radical resections could be performed in most patients who underwent CEA-guided second-look laparotomy. Our own experience confirmed a survival benefit for patients whose metastases were disclosed by CEA determinations compared to patients with metastases diagnosed by other methods (Hohenberger et al. 1994; Quentmeier et al. 1990). A meta-analysis of various follow-up programs after resection of colorectal cancer demonstrated an improved survival of 9% in the patients in the programs with CEA determinations (Bruinvels et al. 1994).

Another potential role of CEA is in monitoring the response to treatment of patients with recurrent or metastatic disease. If adjuvant therapy is performed postoperatively, increasing CEA levels may indicate recurrent disease. More than 80% of patients with colorectal cancer have elevated serum CEA concentrations. It has been demonstrated that a drop in the CEA level during chemotherapy is associated with improved survival of the patients (Allen Mersh et al. 1987). This probably reflects destruction of the tumor by the treatment. On the other hand, in a study of 33 patients who received therapy for metastatic disease, increasing CEA levels were seen in patients with progressive disease confirmed by computed tomography (Ward et al. 1993).

Conclusions

Currently CEA must be considered as the marker of choice for colorectal cancer. However, CEA is not recommended for use in screening for colorectal cancer. Concentrations of this tumor marker should be determined preoperatively because they can assist staging, treatment planning, and postoperative monitoring of adjuvant therapy. Postoperatively CEA testing should be performed every 2-3 months. An elevated or increasing CEA level, if confirmed by retesting, warrants further evaluation of the patient for local recurrence or metastatic disease. However, present data do not justify the use of CEA alone for postoperative follow-up and monitoring of adjuvant therapy. Molecular genetic techniques are increasingly used for risk assessment and identification of hereditary familial colorectal cancer syndromes. Several genetic alterations associated with colorectal cancer, including alterations of *p53* n-*myc*, and k-*ras*, have been identified. The value of these genetic markers compared to conventional staging has not yet been established. One of the most exciting advances in the understanding and prevention of colorectal cancer was the characterization of the APC gene in patients with FAP. It seems likely that in the future molecular genetic techniques will gain major importance in the detection and treatment of colorectal cancer and may contribute substantially to improved patient outcome.

References

Aaltonen LA, Peltomaki P (1994) Genes involved in hereditary nonpolyposis colorectal carcinoma. Anticancer Res 14:1657-1660

Allen Mersh TG, Kemeny N, Niedzwiecki D, Shurgot B, Daly JM (1987) Significance of a fall in serum CEA concentration in patients treated with cytotoxic chemotherapy for disseminated colorectal cancer. Gut 28:1625-1629

ASCO (1996) Clinical practice guidelines for the use of tumor markers in breast and colorectal cancer. Adopted on May 17, 1996 by the American Society of Clinical Oncology. J Clin Oncol 14:2843-2877

Baigrie RJ, Berry AR (1994) Management of advanced rectal cancer. Br J Surg 81:343-352

Benhattar J, Losi L, Chaubert P, Givel JC, Costa J (1993) Prognostic significance of K-*ras* mutations in colorectal carcinoma. Gastroenterology 104:1044-1048

Bodmer WF, Bailey CJ, Bodmer J, Bussey HJ, Ellis A, Gorman P, et al (1987) Localization of the gene for familial adenomatous polyposis on chromosome 5. Nature 328:614-616

Boland CR, Troncale FJ (1984) Familial colonic cancer without antecedent polyposis. Ann Intern Med 100:700-701

Bruinvels DJ, Stiggelbout AM, Kievit J, van Houwelingen HC, Habbema JD, van de Velde CJ (1994) Follow-up of patients with colorectal cancer. A meta-analysis. Ann Surg 219:174-182

Cohen AM, Minsky BD, Schilsky RL (1997) Cancer of the colon. In: De Vita VT, Hellmann S, Rosenberg SA (eds) Principles and practice of oncology, Vol. 1, Lippincott-Raven, Philadelphia, 88:1144-1197

Costanza ME, Das S, Nathanson L, Rule A, Schwartz RS (1974) Proceedings: Carcinoembryonic antigen. Report of a screening study. Cancer 33:583-590

Cummings KM, Michalek A, Tidings J, Herrera L, Mettlin C (1986) Results of a public screening program for colorectal cancer. N Y State J Med 86:68-72

Fishel R, Lescoe MK, Rao MR, Copeland NG, Jenkins NA, Garber J, et al (1994) The human mutator gene homolog MSH2 and its association with hereditary nonpolyposis colon cancer. Cell 77:167

Fletcher RH (1986) Carcinoembryonic antigen. Ann Intern Med 104:66-73

Gerhard M, Juhl H, Kalthoff H, Schreiber HW, Wagener C, Neumaier M (1994) Specific detection of carcinoembryonic antigen-expressing tumor cells in bone marrow aspirates by polymerase chain reaction. J Clin Oncol 12:725-729

Hohenberger P, Schlag P, Gerneth T, Herfarth C (1994) Pre- and postoperative carcinoembryonic antigen determination in hepatic resection fo colorectal metastases. Ann Surg 219:135-143

Jen J, Kim H, Piantadosi S, Liu ZF, Levitt RC, Sistonen P, et al (1994) Allelic loss of chromosome 18q and prognosis in colorectal cancer. N Engl J Med 331:213-221

Kern SE, Pietenpol JA, Thiagalingam S, Seymour A, Kinzler KW, Vogelstein B (1992) Oncogenic forms of p53 inhibit p53-regulated gene expression. Science 256:827-830

Kinzler KW, Nilbert MC, Vogelstein B, Bryan TM, Levy DB, Smith KJ, et al (1991) Identification of a gene located at chromosome 5q21 that is mutated in colorectal cancers. Science 251:1366-1370

Laurent-Puig P, Olschwang P, Delattre O, Remvikos Y, Asselain B, Melot T, et al (1992) Survival and acquired genetic alterations in colorectal cancer. Gastroenterology 102:1136-1141

Lynch HT, Smyrk TC, Watson P, Lanspa SJ, Lynch JF, Lynch PM, et al (1993) Genetics, natural history, tumor spectrum, and pathology of hereditary nonpolyposis colorectal cancer: an update review. Gastroenterology 104:1535-1549

Mandel JS, Bond JH, Church TR, Snover DC, Bradley GM, Schumann LM, Ederer F (1993) Reducing mortality from colorectal cancer by screening for fecal occult blood. Minnesota Colon Cancer Control Study. N Engl J Med 328:1365-1371

Morris JB, Stellato TA, Guy BB, Gordon NH, Berger NA (1991) A critical analysis of the largest reported mass fecal occult blood screening program in the United States. Am J Surg 161:101-105

Neumaier M, Gerhard M, Wagener C (1995) Diagnosis of micrometastases by the amplification of tissue-specific genes. Gene 159:43-47

Quentmeier A, Schlag P, Smok M, Herfarth C (1990) Re-operation for recurrent colorectal cancer: the importance of early diagnosis for resectability and survival. Eur J Surg Oncol 16:319-325

Schlag PM, Hünerbein M, Hohenberger P (1996) Surgical resection of metastatic cancer to the liver. Acta Chir Austriaca 28:27-32

Sener SF, Imperato JP, Chmiel J, Fremgen A, Sylvester J (1989) The use of cancer registry data to study preoperative carcinoembryonic antigen level as an indicator of survival in colorectal cancer. CA Cancer J Clin 39:50-57

Sidransky D, Tokino T, Hamilton SR, Kinzler KW, Levin B, Frost P, Vogelstein B (1992) Identification of ras oncogene mutations in the stool of patients with curable colorectal tumors. Science 256:102-105

Steele G Jr, Ellenberg S, Ramming K, O'Connell M, Moertel C, Lessner H, et al (1982) CEA monitoring among patients in multi-institutional adjuvant GI therapy protocols. Ann Surg 196:162-169

Stevens DP, Mackay IR, Cullen KJ (1975) Carcinoembryonic antigen in an unselected elderly population: a four year follow up. Br J Cancer 32:147-151

Stipa S, Nicolanti V, Botti C, Cosimelli M, Mannella E, Stipa F, et al (1991) Local recurrence after curative resection for colorectal cancer: frequency, risk factors and treatment. J Surg Oncol Suppl 2:155-160

Vogelstein B, Fearon ER, Hamilton SR, Kern SE, Preisinger AC, Leppert M, et al (1988) Genetic alterations during colorectal-tumor development. N Engl J Med 319:525-532

Vukasin AP, Ballantyne GH, Flannery JT, Lerner E, Modlin IM (1990) Increasing incidence of cecal and sigmoid carcinoma. Data from the Connecticut Tumor Registry. Cancer 66:2442-2449

Wagner C (1996) Onkologie 2000: die Sicht des klinischen Laboratoriumsmediziners. Onkologe 2:34-38

Ward U, Pimrose JN, Finan PJ, Perren TJ, Selby P, Purves DA, Cooper EH (1993) The use of tumor markers CEA, CA-195 and CA242 in evaluating the response to chemotherapy in patients with advanced colorectal cancer. Br J Cancer 67:1132-1135

Wolmark N, Fisher B, Wiand HS, Henry RS, Lerner H, Legault Poisson S, et al (1984) The prognostic significance of preoperative carcinoembryonic antigen levels in colorectal cancer. Results from NSABP (National Surgical Adjuvant Breast and Bowel Project) clinical trials. Ann Surg 199:375-382

Surgical Strategy

Possibilities of Extensive Surgery

W. Hohenberger, K. E. Matzel, and U. Stadelmaier

Department of Surgery, University Hospital, University of Erlangen-Nürnberg
Krankenhausstr. 12, 91054 Erlangen, Germany

Abstract

Advances in surgical technique and knowledge of tumor biology have led to an algorithm of surgical treatment of rectal cancer, which offers three options: transanal local excision, sphincter-saving procedures (low anterior resection and, recently, intersphincteric abdomino-peranal resection), and abdomino-perineal resection of the rectum. The choice of operative procedure aiming to fulfill both oncological and functional criteria is determined by the anatomic location of the tumor, the tumor differentiation, the depth of tumor invasion, and preoperative anal sphincter function. Following the algorithm of treatment, a clear decrease can be noted during recent years in the number of abdomino-perineal resections and a shift towards sphincter-sparing procedures, without jeopardizing long-term survival. Although anal sphincter morphology can usually be maintained, preserving the anal sphincter does not necessarily mean preserving the sphincter function. The functional outcome must be judged by objective, measurable parameters and by the impact of operative sequelae on quality of life and its acceptance by the patient. Future work must focus on further improving long-term survival and functional outcome.

Technical advances (Goligher et al. 1979; Heald 1980) and an improved understanding of tumor biology, especially metastatic behavior, have resulted in varied strategies for the operative treatment of rectal cancer. The common aims of these techniques are local control, avoidance of local recurrence, and – while still satisfying oncologic requirements – preservation of the anal sphincter.

Until the 1970s, abdominoperineal excision was the treatment of choice. Subsequently, a shift toward anterior and low anterior resection of the rectum took place. Initially these procedures were limited to the treatment of tumors in the upper and mid rectum (Table 1) (Gall and Hermanek 1992), but the indication for anterior resection was later extended to tumors of the lower rectum (Table 2) (Hohenberger and Hermanek 1992).

Table 1. Curative resection for rectal cancer: historical perspective

Operation:	1969–1977 (n=605)	1978–1983 (n=624)	1984–1988 (n=521)
LAR	255 (42.1%)	344 (53.5%)	318 (61.0%)
APR	323 (53.4%)	213 (34.1%)	155 (29.8%)

LAR, low anterior resection; APR, abdomino-perineal resection. Date from Gall and Hermanek (1992)

Table 2. Operative procedure in relation to tumor location

	Upper rectum LAR	Upper rectum APR	Mid rectum LAR	Mid rectum APR	Lower rectum LAR	Lower rectum APR
1969–1978	n=128 92.2%	7.8%	n=178 72.7%	27.3%	n=242 22.0%	78.0%
1979–1985	n=156 95.5%	4.5%	n=226 88.3%*	12.7%	n=219 14.7%	85.3%

* $p<0.01$
Data from Hohenberger and Hermanek (1992)

With the increasing use of sphincter-sparing procedures, an increase in local recurrence, up to 43%, was observed (Gall 1984). This finding led to a recommendation for a distal clearance margin of at least 3 cm in anterior resection, the 3 cm to be measured on the harvested, fresh, unstretched specimen (equaling an intraoperative distal margin of approximately 5 cm) (Hermanek et al. 1985; Hohenberger and Hermanek 1989); the mesorectum was not to be excised completely, but coning of the excised mesorectum was to be avoided.

This requirement still holds true for carcinomas of the upper third of the rectum, but for tumors of the mid and lower rectum this oncologic postulate conflicted with the effort to spare the anal sphincter, which in some patients would make anterior resection become unacceptable.

The further development of extended but sphincter-saving surgical procedures was based on the following principles:
- Complete excision of the mesorectum is essential for local control of the tumor and avoidance of local recurrence (Heald et al. 1982; Heald and Ryall 1986; Scott et al. 1995).
- Depending on stage and differentiation, for the majority of tumors a distal clearance margin of 1 cm in situ is acceptable (Hermanek and Kimpfinger 1994).
- Partial resection of the internal anal sphincter reduces sphincter function, but does not necessarily result in fecal incontinence (Schiessel et al. 1986).
- By identifying tumors with a low risk of lymphatic metastasis, local procedures with a small safety margin can be acceptable (Gall 1991).

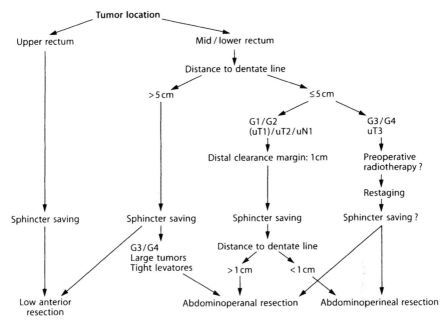

Fig. 1. Algorithm for nonlocal surgical treatment of rectal cancer. G, Histological grading; uT, uN, endosonographic tumor and lymph node staging

The oncologic acceptability of limiting the distal safety margin to 1 cm in low-grade tumors, and the acceptability of partial removal of the internal anal sphincter (acceptable, that is, with regard to functional outcome), led to the development of the intersphincteric abdominoperanal resection (Schiessel et al. 1986). Abdominoperineal excision became avoidable in another 5%–10% of patients with cancer of the lower rectum.

Thus, the options for surgical treatment of rectal cancer are three-fold: transanal local excision; sphincter-saving procedures (low anterior resection and abdominoperanal resection); and abdominoperineal resection (Hohenberger et al. 1992). Complete mesorectal excision, providing adequate circumferential safety margins, is mandatory in tumors of the mid and lower rectum that require a radical procedure (Fiedling et al. 1991).

If local or limited procedures are excluded, the operative strategy for resection follows an algorithm (Fig. 1) that is determined by oncologic and functional criteria:
- The location of the tumor and its relation to the dentate line
- Tumor differentiation
- The depth of tumor invasion
- Preoperative anal sphincter function (patients with reduced sphincter function or preexisting fecal incontinence are not suited to abdominoperanal resection)

Table 3. Sphincter-saving procedures: Erlangen 1990–1994

	Mid rectum ($n=169$)	Lower rectum ($n=196$)
Local excision	3 (1.8%)	14 (7.1%)
Tubular resection	1 (0.6%)	1 (0.5%)
Posterior rectotomy		1 (0.5%)
Low anterior resection	157 (92.9%)	77 (39.3%)
Intersphincteric resection		10 (5.1%)
Abdominoperineal resection	8 (4.7%)	93 (47.4%)

Table 4. Local recurrence rate: Erlangen 1990–1994 [a]

Tumor location	Low anterior resection ($n=156$)	Abdominoperineal resection ($n=55$)
Upper rectum ($n=45$)	2/45 (4%)	–
Mid rectum ($n=77$)	7/74 (10%)	0/3
Lower rectum ($n=89$)	6/37 (16%)	6/52 (12%)

[a] Postoperative mortality or follow up <2 years excluded

Preoperative radiation therapy may enable sphincter-saving procedures in some patients in whom abdominoperineal excision would otherwise be required.

From June 1992 to December 1994, this algorithm was applied prospectively in a group of 60 patients in Regensburg, Germany. In 75% of 56 patients who underwent surgery, sphincter-saving procedures were carried out: in 62.5% low anterior resection, in 7% intersphincteric resection, and in 5.5% transanal local excision.

In Erlangen, retrospective analysis revealed that between 1990 and 1994 sphincter preservation was possible in 95.3% of patients with tumor manifestation in the mid rectum and in 52.6% with cancer of the lower rectum (Table 3).

The different surgical approaches satisfy oncologic requirements and allow preservation of the sphincter. Although the recurrence rate after low anterior resection is known (Table 4), local recurrence over the long term in patients treated by the new intersphincteric procedure has yet to be assessed. Short-term results are promising: among 16 patients with a median follow-up of 600 days, one local recurrence has been noted.

In this treatment algorithm, sphincter preservation is secondary to local tumor control. In addition to causing intraoperative trauma, the operative procedures result in major changes to the anatomy and physiologic integrity of the anorectal organ of continence. Moreover, postoperative changes in stool consistency pose a challenge to fecal continence. Thus, it remains debatable whether preservation of the anal sphincter results in preservation of sphincter function.

Table 5. Clinical results after rectum resection

	Level of anastomosis (cm)			
	≤3	3–6	7–9	≥10
No. of patients	3	12	20	13
Leakage overall	3 (100%)	9 (75.0%)	9 (45.0%)	5 (38.5%)
Incontinence overall	3 (100%)	5 (41.7%)	5 (25.0%)	3 (23.1%)
Reduced ability to defer stool	3 (100%)	6 (50.0%)	6 (30.0%)	2 (15.2%)
Regular use of pads	3 (100%)	6 (50.0%)	6 (30.0%)	0
Anal soreness	3 (100%)	6 (50.0%)	2 (10.0%)*	1 (7.7%)

* $P<0.05$

Table 6. Manometric data after rectum resection

	Level of anastomosis (cm)				
	≤3	3–6	7–9	≥10	Norm
Resting pressure (mmHg)	32.33	32.33	37.75	41.92	>40
Maximal tolerable volume (ml)	50.00	50.83	77.00	171.46*	>200
Compliance (ml/mmHg)	2.65	3.08	3.65	6.53*	6–8

* $P<0.002$

For these reasons, 48 patients who had undergone low anterior resection in Erlangen in 1993 and 1994 were studied (Matzel et al. 1996). Clinical outcome and anorectal physiologic function were assessed. In all cases a potentially curative resection (R0) was performed. None of the patients had pre- or postoperative radiation therapy. Intestinal continuity was restored with straight reconstruction. Median follow-up was 18 months.

Overall, a trend was seen toward increased functional impairment with lower levels of anastomosis, 54% being affected (Table 5). Among patients with anastomoses above or at 10 cm ($n=13$), continence was impaired in 39%; with anastomoses at between 7 and 9 cm ($n=20$), impairment occurred in 46%; for between 4 and 6 cm ($n=12$), it was noted in 75%; and when the anastomosis was located at below 3 cm ($n=3$), impairment occurred in 100%. Reduced continence was mainly the result of an inability to defer the urge to void. Anal soreness and the need for regular use of sanitary pads lent clinical support to these findings.

Impairment of fecal continence was mainly due to reduced function of the neoreservoir, and to a lesser extent from impaired sphincter function (Table 6). Anal resting pressure was only slightly reduced, showing greater impairment with lower levels of anastomosis. Squeeze pressure was not affected. Compliance and maximal tolerable volume were clearly reduced when the anastomoses were located at between 3 and 9 cm (compliance: anastomotic level $\geqslant 10$ cm, 6.53 ml/mmHg; 7-9 cm, 3.65 ml/mmHg; 4-6 cm, 3.08 ml/mmHg; $\leqslant 3$ cm, 2.65 ml/mmHg. Maximal tolerable volume: anastomotic level $\geqslant 10$ cm, 171 ml; 7-9 cm, 77 ml; 4-6 cm, 51 ml; $\leqslant 3$ cm: 50 ml). In only one of the patients to whom the algorithm was applied prospectively did a permanent colostomy become necessary owing to unacceptable fecal incontinence.

Even though continence is reduced after low anterior and intersphincteric resection, resulting potentially in reduced quality of life, most patients reported satisfaction with the overall postoperative result: 82% of those studied with regard to continence would choose to undergo the operation again. Impaired function seems to be more acceptable than a permanent colostomy.

Even though preservation of the anal sphincter in sphincter-sparing rectal resection does not necessarily mean preservation of sphincteric function, final judgment of the operative outcome must be based on objective measurable parameters and acceptance of the functional result by the patient. On the other hand, as reduced continence correlates highly with decreased neorectal compliance, it should be investigated whether increasing compliance by colonic pouch procedures will improve fecal continence.

References

Fiedling LP, Arsenault PA, Chapuis PH, Dent O, Catright B, Hardcastle JD, Hermanek P, Jass JR, Newland RC (1991) Clinico-pathological staging for colorectal cancer: an international documentation system (IDS) and an international comprehensive anatomical terminology (ICAT). J Gastroenterol Hepatol 6:325-344

Gall FP (1984) Indikationswandel beim kolorektalen Karzinom. In: Gall FP, Hohenberger W (eds) Aktuelle Chirurgie. Indikationen gestern und heute. Urban & Schwarzenberg, Munich, pp 78-83

Gall FP (1991) Cancer of the rectum - local excision. Int J Colorectal Dis 6:84-85

Gall FP, Hermanek P (1992) Wandel und derzeitiger Stand der chirurgischen Behandlung des colorectalen Carcinoms. Chirurg 63:227-234

Goligher JC, Lee PWR, Macfie J et al (1979) Experiences with the Russian model 249 suture gun for anastomosis of the rectum. Surg Gynaecol Obstet 148:517-524

Heald RJ (1980) Towards fewer colostomies - the impact of circular stapling devices on surgery of rectal cancer in a district hospital. Br J Surg 60:198-200

Heald RJ, Ryall RD (1986) Recurrence and survival after total mesorectal excision for rectal cancer. Lancet 1479-1482

Heald RJ, Husband EM, Ryall, RDH (1982) The mesorectum in rectal cancer surgery - the clue to pelvic recurrence? Br J Surg 69:613-616

Hermanek P, Gall FP, Guggenmoos-Holzmann I, Altendorf A (1985) Pathogenesis of local recurrence after surgical treatment of rectal carcinoma. Dig Surg 2:7-14

Hermanek P, Kimpfinger M (1994) Sphinktererhaltende radikale Resektion des Rektum-Karzinoms aus der Sicht der Pathologie. Acta Chir Austriaca 26:122-130

Hohenberger W, Hermanek, P (1989) Weite des aboralen Sicherheitsabstandes bei anteriorer Rektumresektion. In: Gall FP, Zirngibl H, Hermanek P (eds) Das kolorektale Karzinom. Zuckschwerdt, Munich, pp 161-174

Hohenberger W, Hermanek P Jr, Hermanek P, Gall FP (1992) Decision-making in curative rectum carcinoma surgery. Oncology 15:209-220

Matzel KE, Stadelmaier U, Dünne A, Hohenberger W (1996) Impact of level of anastomosis on continence after colorectal and coloanal reconstruction following resection for cancer. Dis Colon Rectum 39:A12

Scott N, Jackson P, Al-Jaberi T, Dixon MF, Quirke P, Finan PJ (1995) Total mesorectal excision and local recurrence: a study of tumour spread in the mesorectum distal to rectal cancer. Br J Surg 82:1031-1033

Schiessel R, Wunderlich M, Waneck R (1986) Ergebnisse der coloanalen Anastomose bei tiefsitzenden Tumoren des Rectums. Chirurg 57:791-796

Total Mesorectal Excision for Cancer of the Rectum

P. Aeberhard and F. Fasolini

Department of Surgery, Cantonal Hospital, 5001 Aarau, Switzerland

Abstract

The concept of total mesorectal excision (TME) was first described by R.J. Heald in 1982 as a radical cancer operation based on the anatomy of fascial planes and fibrous spaces of the pelvis. The ampulla recti is invested by a fascia propria which is a part of the visceral pelvic fascia. The fascia propria is separated from the parietal pelvic fascia by the pelvirectal fibrous space, which is a compartment of the subperitoneal space of the pelvis. The lateral ligaments of the rectum divides the pelvirectal space into a prerectal and a retrorectal part. TME is defined as the resection of the rectum with its surrounding fatty and lymphatic tissue contained within the visceral sheet of the pelvic fascia. The dissection proceeds in the nearly avascular cleavage plane between the visceral and the parietal fascial sheets, allowing maximal protection of the hypogastric nerves and the inferior hypogastric plexus. Continuity of the prerectal and retrorectal parts of the field of dissection is established by dividing the lateral ligaments of the rectum slightly inside the point where they swing away from the parietal fascia of the pelvic side wall. By following this plane of dissection it is possible to achieve en bloc excision of the total mass of perirectal lymphatic and fatty tissue down to the pelvic floor.

The concept of total mesorectal excision was introduced by R.J. Heald et al. 1982. These authors presented evidence suggesting that total excision of the mesorectum during resection for rectal cancer reduces the risk of local tumor recurrence. They recommended that when performing a low anterior resection the mesorectum should not be transected at the level of transection of the rectum, but rather excised totally down to its end, which lies at the point of fusion of the parietal and visceral sheets of the pelvic fascia at the level of the tip of the coccyx. R.J. Heald, later (1988) elaborated on the concept by defining the "holy plane" of rectal surgery, describing total mesorectal excision as resection of the rectum together with the fatty and lymphatic tissue contained within the visceral sheet of the pelvic fascia. Köckerling and Gall (1994) published a very clear and detailed description of the anatomical basis and technical details of the operation. Their publication, together with

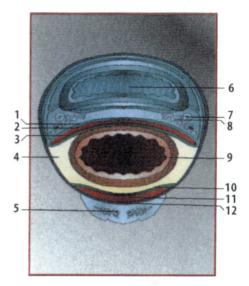

Fig. 1. *1,* Vesical fascia (continuing caudally into Denonvillier's fascia); *2,* praerectal fibrous space; *3, 10,* fascia propria of rectum; *4,* perirectal fatty tissue; *5,* sacrum; *6,* bladder; *7,* ureter; *8,* seminal vesicle; *9,* rectum; *11,* retrorectal fibrous space; *12,* Waldeyer's fascia (part of parietal pelvic fascia). (Illustration by F. Fasolini)

the essentials of the relevant anatomy as published in the classical work Praktische Anatomie edited by Lanz and Wachsmuth (Lierse et al. 1984) and in the Ciba Atlas of medical illustrations (Netter 1962), forms the basis for the terminology and illustrations used in the present chapter.

This chapter is about a video presented at the Berlin Meeting in 1996.[1] The aim of the video was to explain the anatomical basis and the technical steps to follow when performing a total mesorectal excision for cancer of the midrectum, and the present paper chapter has the same aim. We will not enter into a discussion of the oncological value of the procedure, which has been covered by L. P. Fielding (1993).

The ampulla recti is invested by a *fascia propria* which is a part of the *visceral pelvic fascia*. The fascia propria is separated from the *parietal pelvic fascia* by the *pelvirectal fibrous space*, a compartment of the subperitoneal space of the pelvis. The *lateral ligaments* divide the pelvirectal space into a prerectal and a retrorectal part. The plane of dissection which is followed in total mesorectal excision is the nearly avascular cleavage plane between the visceral and parietal fascial sheets (Fig. 1).

The abdomen is opened either by a long midline incision from the xiphisternum to the pubis or a lower midline incision extended obliquely to the left costal margin. Mobilization of the splenic flexure is an essential step which ensures sufficient mobility of the proximal bowel for construction of a tension-free low rectal anastomosis. The entire left hemicolon is lifted off the *prerenal fascia of Gerota*. The inferior mesenteric vein is ligated and trans-

---

[1] The video is available through the Videothek SGL, Postfach, CH-8134 Adliswi

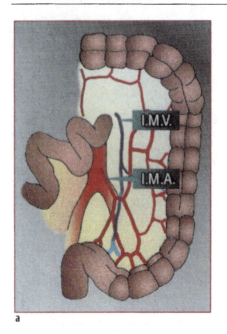 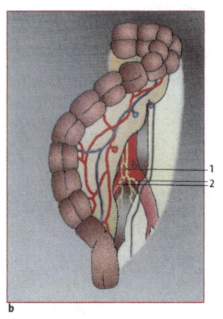

Fig. 2. a *IMA*, Inferior mesenteric artery; *IMV*, inferior mesenteric vein. **b** *1*, Superior hypogastric plexus; *2*, right and left hypogastric nerve. (Illustration by F. Fasolini)

ected at the lower border of the pancreas, and the inferior mesenteric artery is secured and cut at its origin from the aorta (Fig. 2). The correct cleavage plane in the retrorectal fibrous space is automatically entered when dissection along Gerota's fascia is continued caudally over the pelvic brim on to *Waldeyer's fascia*, which is the downward continuation of Gerota's fascia and constitutes the dorsal part of the parietal fascia of the pelvis (Crapp and Cuthbertson 1974). While proceeding along this fascial plane in front of the aorta and common iliac arteries, the *superior hypogastric plexus* and its division into the right and left *hypogastric nerves* can be identified shining through the fascial covering and securely preserved. After entering the *retrorectal fibrous space* the dissection is continued caudally and forwards around the pelvic side wall. Anteriorly the peritoneum is opened slightly in front of the peritoneal reflection and the *prerectal fibrous space* entered. This dissection should be started in the midline and continued laterally only after identification of the correct plane of dissection along *Denonvillier's fascia*. The *lateral ligaments* of the rectum are then divided following a plane which is slightly inside the parietal fascia of the pelvic side wall (Fig. 3a). The ligaments must be divided stepwise, using coagulation and hemostatic clips. Forceful traction must be avoided, as this tends to tear the nerves of the *inferior hypogastric plexus* off the pelvic side wall, with the risk of damaging them. The dorsal dissection is completed by cutting through the fibrous strands of the rectosacral fascia down to the point of fusion with the fascia propria of

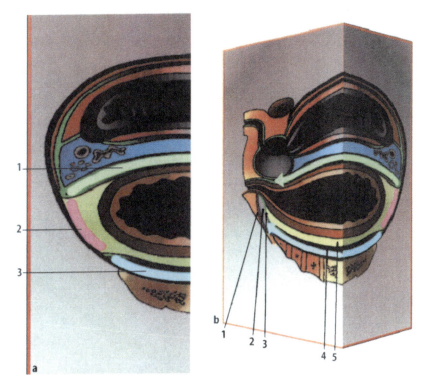

Fig. 3. a *1, Green,* prerectal fibrous space; *2, red,* plane of transection of lateral ligament; *3, blue,* retrorectal fibrous space. **b** Anterior and posterior dissection in the perirectal fibrous space down to the pelvic floor. *1,* Rectococcygeus muscle; *2,* infrarectal space; *3,* rectosacral fascia; *4,* retrorectal fibrons space; *5,* mesorectum

the rectum, which is at the level of the tip of the coccyx and marks the lower end of the mesorectum. With the division of the *rectosacral fascia,* the *infrarectal space* has been entered (Fig. 3b), and from this point down to the anorectal junction, the rectum is a tube of muscle devoid of fatty tissue. Total mesorectal excision allows distal transection of the rectum at any point from about 4 cm above the levators down to the anorectal junction.

The dorsal side of a good specimen of total mesorectal excision must have a typical bilobed appearance. These two lobes of fatty tissue are a mold of the paired concavities created by the levator ani muscles.

References

Crapp AR, Cuthbertson AM (1974) William Waldeyer and the rectosacral fascia. Surg Gynecol Obstet 138:252–256
Fielding LP (1993) Mesorectal excision for rectal cancer. Lancet 341:471–472
Heald RJ (1988) The "holy plane" of rectal surgery. J R Soc Med 81:503–508

Heald RJ, Husband EM, Ryall RDH (1982) The mesorectum in rectal cancer surgery – the clue to pelvic recurrence? Br J Surg 69:613–616

Köckerling F, Gall FP (1994) Chirurgische Standards beim Rectumcarcinom. Chirurg 65:593–603

Lierse W, Frohmüller H, Stelzner F, Stegner HE (1984) Becken. In: von Lanz T, Wachsmuth W, Lang J (Hrsg) Praktische Anatomie, Bd 2/Teil 8A. Springer, Berlin Heidelberg New York

Netter FH (1962) Nervous system. In: The Ciba collection of medical illustrations, vol 1. CIBA

Radical Surgery for Extensive Rectal Cancer: Is It Worthwhile?

F. L. Moffat, Jr.[1], and R. E. Falk[2]

[1] Division of Oncology, Department of Surgery, University of Miami School of Medicine, Sylvester Comprehensive Cancer Center, Surgical Oncology (310T), Rm. 3550, 1475 N.W. 12th Av., Miami, FL 33136, USA
[2] University of Toronto Department of Surgery, Division of General Surgery, Toronto General Hospital, Toronto, Ontario, Canada

Abstract

In a small proportion of patients with extensive primary or locally recurrent rectal cancer, disease remains confined to the pelvis for a prolonged period. Symptoms are highly prejudicial to quality of life and often refractory to treatment short of extirpative surgery. Cure requires en bloc excision of all involved pelvic viscera with tumor-free margins. The pelvic exenterations (PE) are the most radical operations for rectal cancer. PE carries a high risk of perioperative morbidity and mortality, and has profound functional, psychological, and psychosexual implications for patients. Careful preoperative counseling regarding surgical risks and the impact of PE on body function and image is indispensable; the patient's consent must be truly informed. Patients with major medical or psychiatric/emotional comorbidity and those who are mentally incompetent are not candidates. Tenesmus and central pelvic/perineal pain are amenable to PE whereas radicular pain is not; sciatica and lower extremity lymphedema portend unresectability. Extrapelvic disease should be excluded preoperatively. While invaded sacrum can be resected en bloc with involved viscera (sacropelvic exenteration), fixity of tumor to the pelvic sidewall(s) in nonirradiated patients almost invariably implies unresectability. Other contraindications to PE include invasion of the proximal (S1 or higher) lumbosacral spine or lumbosacral plexus/sciatic nerves, ureteric obstruction proximal to the ureterovesical junctions, and encasement of the external or common iliac vessels by tumor. PE for advanced primary rectal carcinoma yields 5-year survival of over 40%; when performed for recurrent disease, long-term salvage rates are not as high. While radical surgery is rarely indicated for palliation, PE in carefully selected (good performance status and life expectancy, complete excision of all gross disease) incurable patients results in abrogation of disabling symptoms and reasonable intervals of high-quality survival.

Introduction

While increasingly uncommon, extensive primary or locoregionally recurrent rectal adenocarcinomas involving multiple pelvic structures continue to challenge oncologists of all disciplines. In a small proportion of rectal cancer patients, disease remains confined to the pelvis for a prolonged period of time, metastasizing late or not at all (Eckhauser et al. 1979; Falk et al. 1985). In patients with rectal cancer recurrence in the pelvis, most symptoms, morbidity, and up to 75% of cancer-related mortality can be attributed to the recurrent pelvic disease, even in those in whom metastasis beyond the pelvis has occurred (Moffat et al. 1994b).

Patients with extensive rectal cancer are at risk of a particularly miserable demise if inadequately treated, and often have little or no "quality" in their lives to speak of. Many of these individuals experience unremitting central pelvic/perineal pain, tenesmus, and/or urinary urgency refractory to all non-surgical interventions including advanced techniques in cancer pain management. These severe, disabling pain syndromes may be compounded by bleeding or malodorous perineal discharge from necrotic, infected tumor and urinary or intestinal fistulae; patients in whom these manifestations develop often become social pariahs even to their own families and attending medical and nursing personnel.

While locoregionally advanced primary rectal cancers are susceptible to preoperative downstaging using cytotoxic chemotherapy and irradiation, cure of these bulky tumors is rarely realized, and symptoms are poorly or only transiently alleviated if treatment does not include aggressive surgery. Extensive recurrent rectal cancer is even less likely to be controlled by less-than-radical surgery. Radical extirpative pelvic operations continue to be essential, albeit infrequently indicated, options in the surgical oncologist's armamentarium for adenocarcinoma of the rectum.

The discussion which follows is focused on the use of exenterative pelvic operations in patients with extensive primary and recurrent rectal cancer. Pelvic exenteration, and especially total pelvic exenteration, is the most extreme example of extirpative surgery for pelvic neoplasia. These operations therefore throw into bold relief the issues and controversies surrounding the use of radical pelvic surgery for rectal cancer. Clinical experience with pelvic exenteration exemplifies the benefits and problems attendant, to a comparable or lesser degree, on other radical rectal cancer operations.

Patient Selection and Preoperative Evaluation

Exenterative pelvic surgery carries a high risk of morbidity and mortality, and is very demanding of the surgeon and hospital resources. Moreover, the functional and psychological consequences of these radical operations are enormous.

The magnitude of the physiological stress and operative risks associated with exenterative surgery are prohibitive for patients with major, irremediable medical comorbidity. However, chronological age by itself should not be a major factor in selection of patients for exenterative pelvic surgery.

The functional, psychological, and psychosexual effects of exenteration are profound. Such surgery should not be performed on patients with mental or emotional illnesses, or on mentally incompetent individuals. Preoperative education and counseling regarding the proposed surgery and its associated risks and impact on body functions and image are of critical importance. For prospective patients, these measures expedite the process of coming to terms with the consequences of pelvic evisceration or, in the alternative, afford them the opportunity to arrive at an educated decision to decline the surgery. It is imperative that patients' consent to undergo these procedures be truly informed in every respect.

Preoperative Evaluation for Exenterative Surgery

In addition to assessment of medical and psychological fitness for exenterative surgery, a concerted effort to evaluate resectability and rule out spread of tumor outside the pelvis is required. Careful elucidation of the patient's symptoms is often very revealing. Hematuria, pneumaturia, and other urinary symptoms may signify bladder invasion by recurrent rectal cancer. Many patients with recurrent rectal carcinoma complain of tenesmus or central pelvic and perineal pain, symptoms which are amenable to exenterative procedures. On the other hand, sciatica-like pain is rarely alleviated by salvage surgery, and has an ominous significance. Radicular pain is indicative of tumor infiltration into (and extension along) nerves and perineural lymphatics, a situation in which resection with tumor-free margins is impossible (Ketcham et al. 1970; Deckers et al. 1976; Yeung et al. 1993, 1994).

Examination of the supraclavicular nodes, the inguinal nodes (for distal rectal cancer) and abdomen may reveal evidence of metastasis.

In the absence of a previous history of pelvic irradiation, fixity of tumor to the pelvic sidewall is strong evidence of unresectability. However, sacral invasion by extensive rectal cancer can be resected en bloc in a so-called "sacropelvic" exenteration (Pearlman et al. 1987; Temple and Ketcham 1992; Wanebo et al. 1992, 1994).

In the previously irradiated pelvis, perceived bony fixation of recurrent tumor is frequently the result of treatment-induced fibrosis and not malignant infiltration (Yeung et al. 1993). Definitive evaluation for resectability is usually only possible at laparotomy (Yeung et al. 1993, 1994); computerized tomography (CT), magnetic resonance imaging (MRI), skeletal scintigraphy, and even examination under anaesthesia (EUA) may be uninformative or even misleading in these clinical circumstances.

The presence of lower extremity edema implies malignant obstruction of the external and common iliac venous and/or lymphatic outflow, and as such is an ominous finding. Affected patients are almost never candidates for exenteration because of extent of disease.

Preoperative investigation should include blood chemistry and appropriate tumor markers, chest roentgenogram with thoracic CT if indicated by suspicious findings, abdominopelvic CT, and skeletal scintigraphy. Plain sacral films and MRI may also be of value. Radioimmunoscintigraphy may prove to be a useful adjunct to CT because of its superior sensitivity for detection of transperitoneal and other extrahepatic abdominal disease (Moffat et al. 1994a).

In nonirradiated patients, the extent and mobility of recurrent pelvic disease can be evaluated with considerable accuracy by EUA. Cystoscopic findings of trigonal edema or frank tumor invasion of the bladder confirm the necessity for exenterative surgery. However, the operability of extensive rectal cancer and the extent of surgery required for complete excision of gross disease can often only be determined at laparotomy (Falk et al. 1985; Lindsey et al. 1985, Yeung et al. 1993).

Absolute contraindications to exenteration include proximal (S1 or higher) lumbosacral spine or bony pelvic sidewall invasion, extension of tumor through the sciatic notch or into the lumbosacral plexus or sciatic nerves, bilateral ureteric obstruction above the ureterovesical junctions or external/common iliac vessel encasement by tumor. With few exceptions (vide infra), the presence of distant or abdominal metastases precludes consideration of exenteration. Unilateral upper urinary tract involvement is a relative contraindication to exenteration (Ketcham et al. 1970).

The Operation

Exenterative pelvic surgery places great demands on the patient's physiological reserves and the surgeon's stamina. Reported median blood loss ranges from 3800 to 5000 ml, and operative time from 3.5 to 10 h (Falk et al. 1985; Pearlman et al. 1990; Yeung et al. 1993, 1994). When en bloc resection of portions of the bony pelvis is necessary, blood loss can be prodigious and operative time protracted; in the experience of Wanebo et al. (1992, 1994) with sacropelvic exenteration, median blood loss was 8000 ml and median duration of surgery was 18 h.

At laparotomy, the extent of disease is carefully evaluated with attention to the liver, portal lymph nodes, para-aortic and common iliac lymph nodes, the omentum, and other peritoneal surfaces. Suspicious findings are biopsied to confirm or rule out tumor metastasis.

In evaluating resectability, the pelvic dissection is begun at the point of closest approach of tumor to the bony pelvis (usually the pelvic sidewall) whenever possible. In patients with colorectal cancer recurrence, sacrococcygeal adherence or invasion is often evaluable only after the tumor has been mobilized on each side, especially in the male pelvis. The internal iliac vessels are ligated and divided distal to the superior gluteal artery takeoff, and the distal vessels are included in the operative specimen. The ureters are identified and followed into the true pelvis.

When total or posterior exenteration is planned, ureteric dissection is deferred until tumor resectability is established and the point of ureteric transection determined. The minimum amount of ureteric mobilization necessary for urinary diversion is performed, and the plane of dissection is kept well outside the periureteric vascular plexus. This is especially important in patients with pelvic recurrence in the face of previous radiotherapy and surgery, in whom the ureters are prone to ischemic complications when mobilized and anastomosed to intestinal conduits.

The irradiated pelvis poses special surgical challenges related to fibrotic obliteration of tissue planes and the effects of chronic radiation injury to the small intestine and other abdominal viscera. Pelvic dissection in these individuals is greatly complicated by dense fibrous adhesions. When rectal cancer has recurred between the anterior rectum and adjacent viscera in irradiated patients, we have not infrequently had to resort to the judicious use of an osteotome to accomplish presacral dissection (Falk et al. 1985; Yeung et al. 1993, 1994). Paradoxically, however, operative blood loss, transfusion requirements, and duration of surgery were significantly lower in irradiated than in nonirradiated patients in our experience; the reduced presacral and pelvic sidewall bleeding was presumably due to radiation-induced obliterative endarteritis in pelvic soft tissues.

The distal small bowel in irradiated patients is often adherent in the pelvis, and therefore vulnerable to enterotomy with subsequent fistula or abscess formation. The choice of urinary diversion technique is influenced by a history of previous pelvic radiotherapy and/or findings at surgery compatible with radiation enteritis (vide infra).

In the previously irradiated patient, the distinction between tumor infiltration and treatment-induced fibrosis can be difficult or impossible to make clinically or radiologically, and often confounds the surgeon at laparotomy. Despite concerted efforts to confirm or rule out tumor invasion of contiguous structures, exenterative surgery sometimes results in resection of organs which, because of previous treatment, are densely adherent to the viscus harboring recurrence but are not invaded by the neoplasm. In these and other similar situations, the surgeon is compelled to resect adherent structures, which subsequently prove to be histologically tumor-free, rather than risk dissection into a potentially tumor-infiltrated tissue plane or viscus. Adhesions between a colorectal cancer-bearing viscus and adjacent structures harbor malignant cells 55% –80% of the time (McGlone et al. 1982; Gall et al. 1987). Moreover, dissection into the plane between a colorectal cancer-bearing viscus and an adherent adjacent viscus results in a markedly increased incidence of local recurrence (69% as compared to 18% for en bloc resection; Hunter et al. 1987) and is prejudicial to survival (17%-23% as compared to 49%-61% for en bloc resection at 5 years; Gall et al. 1987; Hunter et al. 1987).

Surgical oncologists are occasionally confronted with a patient in whom, after surgery and radiotherapy for rectal cancer, a large, painful perineal or cloacal sinus develops, with or without an associated pelvic mass. Radiological investigations, EUA, and multiple biopsies fail to confirm tumor recurrence, leaving patient and surgeon to decide whether to proceed with exenteration without proof that recurrent tumor is present. In the final analysis, such a decision is based on the patient's symptomatology, which may be severe and is often refractory to other treatment modalities (Ketcham et al. 1970; Deckers et al. 1976).

There is ongoing controversy concerning the optimal method of urinary diversion in patients undergoing total pelvic exenteration. Ureterosigmoid anastomoses and sigmoid colon conduits have been advocated because an extra anastomosis for restoration of intestinal continuity is avoided. Transverse colon and jejunal conduits employ segments of intestine which are far removed from pelvic radiotherapy portals, thereby reducing the risk of urinary anastomotic leak. The ileal conduit, a popular method of urinary diversion, has been a significant improvement on ureterosigmoidostomy as hyperchloremic acidosis is largely avoided. Continent urinary reservoirs (Pearlman et al. 1990) are recent innovations designed to improve quality of life; some of these confer an additional benefit by helping to fill the pelvic defect. The unresolved debate regarding the optimal method(s) of urinary diversion reflects the dual realities that none of these techniques is clearly superior to the others, and urinary complications continue to figure prominently in the morbidity of pelvic exenteration.

Some surgeons prefer a "two-team" approach to pelvic exenterative surgery (Olsson et al. 1976; Falk et al. 1985; Yeung et al. 1993). Typically, one team performs the resection and pelvic reconstruction and the other undertakes the urinary diversion procedure. Exenteration is a physically taxing operation for surgeons. Moreover, ureteric diversion is a major source of both short- and long-term morbidity and mortality. Involvement of two fresh surgical teams in these major, complication-prone procedures may well have a salutary effect on the incidence of complications.

Management of the pelvic dead space and the perineal wound have been addressed using a variety of surgical approaches. Whereas in the past many surgeons advocated the use of peritoneal flaps, omentum, or synthetic mesh for creation of a "pelvic lid" to exclude the small bowel from the exenterated pelvis, more recently the necessity for closure of the pelvic inlet has been challenged (Ketcham et al. 1970; Falk et al. 1985; Yeung et al. 1993, 1994). Ketcham et al. (1970) observed that obliteration of pelvic dead space to avoid postoperative pelvic sepsis is more important than creation of a pelvic lid. Closure of the pelvic inlet with omentum or peritoneum runs a small risk of small bowel herniation or entrapment with resultant obstruction if defects are left or develop postoperatively. Obliteration of dead space can be accomplished by any (or a combination) of several techniques: careful reapproximation of perineal skin and soft tissues over closed suction drains; the use of gracilis, tensor fascia lata, rectus abdominis, and/or gluteus myocutaneous flaps, or a pedicled omental plug to fill the dead space (Temple and Ketchum 1992); or pelvic urinary enteric conduit (Pearlman et al. 1987) and/or, in female patients, vaginal reconstruction to fill the pelvic defect.

Results of Exenteration for Extensive Rectal Carcinoma

Mortality and Morbidity

Published data on mortality and morbidity for pelvic exenteration in patients with recurrent pelvic tumor are summarized in Table 1. These operations are attended by a substantial risk of perioperative death and complications. Mortality has decreased as advances have been made in nutritional support, anesthesiology, intraoperative monitoring, and postoperative intensive care.

The magnitude of these surgical procedures is further reflected in postoperative hospital stay. Only a minority of patients leave hospital within 14 days of surgery, with median hospital stay ranging from 22 to 38 days. Postoperative complications tend to be both major and multiple; hospital stays in the range of 60–180 days are not unusual for affected patients.

As might be expected, the incidence of complications is formidable, and is higher following exenteration for recurrence than for locoregionally advanced primary cancer (Ketcham et al. 1970; Hafner et al. 1992). Ketcham et al. (1970) clearly documented increased mortality and morbidity when operative time exceeded 7–8 h. Previous irradiation is also a significant risk factor for complications and/or mortality (Ketcham et al. 1970; Hafner et al. 1992). The incidence and multiplicity of early and late complications decrease with the surgeon's experience (Falk et al. 1985; Yeung et al. 1993), and have also been mitigated by improvements in perioperative supportive care.

Table 1. Mortality and morbidity of exenterative surgery for extensive rectal adenocarcinoma

Series	No. of patients	Perioperative mortality (%)	Overall morbidity (%)	No. of complications
Boey (1982)	49	18.4	51	38
Brophy (1994)	35	3	47	6 major, 10 minor
Falk (1985)	45	15.5	58	66 early, 11 late
Hafner (1992)	75	5.3	43	46 major, 28 minor
Kiselow (1967)	43	16	–	–
Jakowatz (1985)	104	8.7	77	69 major, 81 minor
Lopez (1987)	24	20.8	26	12 major
Olsson (1976)	18	6	45	9 early, 5 late
Temple (1992)	9	9	88	2 major, 7 minor
Wanebo (1994)	53	8.6	–	111
Yeung (1993)	50	14	80	39 early, 57 late

In a review of complications associated with exenterative surgery, Pearlman (1994) noted that general or cardiopulmonary complications such as pneumonia, myocardial infarction, or deep venous thrombosis develop in 2%–20% of patients. Wound complications (infection, dehiscence, etc.) can be expected in 16%–30% of patients, and 20%–50% of patients undergoing exenteration will have pelvic or gastrointestinal complications such as bowel obstruction, abscess, enteroperineal fistula, or perineal herniation. The urinary diversion procedure is a source of complications (urosepsis, abscess, anastomotic leak or stricture, or fistula) in 9%–25% of patients.

The most common early complications (intestinal obstruction and fistulae, urinary anastomotic leaks and strictures, and pelvic abscesses) usually require surgical correction. Surgery for post-exenteration fistulae carries a substantial risk of mortality (Moffat et al. 1994b). Unfortunately, the risk of postoperative small bowel obstruction or enteric fistulization has not been eliminated by obliterating the pelvic defect. Pelvic abscesses have occurred less often since attention to obliteration of pelvic dead space has become routine (Ketcham et al. 1970).

Late complications include bowel obstruction, intestinal and urinary fistulae, and obstructive and septic complications related to urinary diversion. Fistulae and obstructions developing months to years after exenteration are frequently due to recurrent tumor. Delayed complications usually require further surgery, and remain a prominent cause of late mortality.

Survival and Recurrence Following Exenteration

Survival data for exenteration with curative intent are given in Table 2. The prospects for cure when exenteration is performed for recurrent rectal carcinoma are less favorable than for extensive primary cancer. With sacropelvic exenteration for recurrence, only 24% of patients survive 5 years (Wanebo et al. 1992).

Kiselow et al. (1967) reported that pelvic nodal involvement results in significantly reduced survival in patients requiring exenterative surgery for rectal cancer. Wanebo et al. (1994) demonstrated in patients undergoing sacropelvic exenteration for recurrent rectal carcinoma that post-exenteration prognosis is adversely affected by microscopically involved surgical margins, pelvic lymph node metastases, the surgical procedure used to excise the original primary cancer (abdominoperineal resection is worse than anterior resection with coloproctostomy), pre-exenteration serum CEA level greater than 10 ng/ml, and the presence of sacral marrow invasion by tumor.

In patients undergoing curative exenteration for rectal cancer, post-exenteration relapse is most often in the pelvis, either alone or in combination with distant metastases. Of the 14 patients reported by Hafner et al. (1991) in whom exenteration for recurrent colorectal cancer eventuated in treatment failure, eight were solitary pelvic or perineal relapses. Boey et al. (1982) reported that, of patients in their series in whom disease recurred following ex-

Table 2. Survival after exenterative surgery with curative intent for extensive rectal carcinoma

Series	No. of patients	Median survival (months)	Five-year survival (%)
Primary rectal cancer			
Boey (1982)	49	–	39
Eckhauser (1979)	12	48	50
Kiselow (1967)	43	–	30
Ledesma (1981)	30	–	43
Lindsey (1985)	32	27	33
Liu (1994)	29	–	56
Lopez (1987)	24	32	42
Takagi (1985)	13	34	38
Williams (1988)	15	38	40
Recurrent rectal cancer			
Hafner (1991)	21	32	33
Yeung (1993)	43	19	10
Wanebo (1994)[a]	47	39	21

[a] Sacropelvic exenteration

enteration, relapse was limited to the pelvis only in 30% and the pelvis plus one or more distant sites in 22%.

Exenteration for Palliation of Incurable Rectal Carcinoma

It is a maxim of clinical oncology that truly radical surgery is contraindicated when cure is not possible. Unfortunately, the surgeon sometimes discovers only after the "point of no return" has been passed in an exenterative operation that rectal cancer cannot be curatively resected. Unintentional palliative exenterations of this nature are unavoidable on occasion.

However, exenteration may be the only recourse for palliation of intractable central pelvic pain, bleeding or draining perineal sinuses, or entero-/uroperineal fistulae in a small, carefully selected group of patients with recurrent, metastatic rectal cancer. Most such patients are "radiation failures," and therefore are usually not eligible for further radiotherapy. Those with chronic tumor- or fistula-related sepsis are poor candidates for palliative chemotherapy. Moreover, cytotoxic chemotherapy is ineffective for bulky, extensive recurrences.

Recent improvements in operative mortality rates may justify the use of exenterative pelvic surgery in selected incurable patients with substantial life expectancy, in whom abrogation of major tumor-related symptoms can reasonably be anticipated provided the pelvis is cleared of all gross tumor (Deckers et al. 1976; Lindsey et al. 1985). Again, the patient must be carefully educated and involved in the decision-making process. The magnitude of the

Table 3. Survival after exenterative surgery with palliative intent for extensive rectal cancer

Series	No. of patients	Median survival (months)
Brophy (1994)	35	20
Deckers (1976)	8	18
Pearlman (1987)	4	9
Wanebo (1994)[a]	6	18
Yeung (1993)	20	10

[a] Sacropelvic exenteration

symptoms to be palliated should be commensurate with the scope of the surgery.

In experienced hands, pelvic exenteration with palliative intent has provided reasonable intervals of high-quality survival (Brophy et al. 1994; Deckers 1976; Olsson et al. 1976; Falk et al. 1985; Lindsey et al. 1985; Wanebo et al. 1992, 1994; Yeung et al. 1993). A case selection policy which categorically excludes *all* incurable patients with resectable, symptomatic pelvic recurrence from consideration for exenterative surgery is probably too restrictive.

Properly selected patients undergoing palliative exenteration survive long enough to enjoy a reasonable symptom-free interval following recovery from surgery. Median survival times in published series of palliative exenterations range from 8.5 to 20 months (Table 3).

Relief of Symptoms and Post-Exenteration Quality of Life

When performed in appropriately selected patients, pelvic exenteration is highly effective in relieving the central pelvic and perineal pain so common among patients with extensive rectal cancer (Ketcham et al. 1970; Deckers et al. 1976; Olsson et al. 1976; Wanebo et al. 1992, 1994; Yeung et al. 1993). A cautionary note is warranted, however; in general, relief of pain should be considered an *added* benefit of exenteration, and should rarely be the primary indication for surgery. It bears repeating that radicular pain is almost never ameliorated by radical surgery. Moreover, effective pain control is attainable only if all gross pelvic disease is resected (Deckers et al. 1976).

Recurrent rectal cancer which is extensive enough to require exenteration almost always causes disabling pain and tenesmus refractory to even large doses of narcotics. Complete relief or marked reduction (i.e., requiring only minor analgesics once or twice a week) of central pelvic pain and tenesmus was experienced in 89% of patients surviving curative exenteration, and in 67% of palliative exenterations, as reported by Yeung et al. (1993). Wanebo et al. (1992) reported relief of pain and other symptoms in 30 of 31 patients undergoing composite pelvic resections; 66% regained their previous lifestyle and 43% returned to work. Similar observations have been made by others

(Ketcham et al. 1970; Deckers et al. 1976; Olsson et al. 1976; Falk et al. 1985; Brophy et al. 1994).

Bleeding or malodorous perineal discharge from necrotic or infected tumor, or urinary and intestinal perineal fistulae, can cause insuperable nursing problems. Rarely, such a situation develops as the sole result of radiation necrosis, and not recurrent tumor (Ketcham et al. 1970; Deckers et al. 1976; Olsson et al. 1976). Pelvic exenteration can be highly effective in these clinical situations; the need for ongoing nursing care is obviated, patients become socially functional and can engage once again in recreational activities and even gainful employment. The results are most gratifying in those in whom the etiology is radiation necrosis (Ketcham et al. 1970), but are also dramatic in properly selected patients with recurrent rectal cancer.

Exenterative surgery exacts a high functional price, but patients for whom these operations are indicated have life-threatening conditions refractory to any other available therapy. Enjoyment of life, social interaction, and economic productivity are difficult or impossible for most patients with extensive rectal adenocarcinoma. Quality of life, as a complicated and multifaceted variable, is perhaps best assessed by questionnaire and interview studies of exenteration patients themselves. Only the patient can appreciate the effects, both beneficial and deleterious, of radical therapeutic intervention on a disease state which itself was often highly prejudicial to the enjoyment of living.

Vera (1981), who studied 19 patients 2–12 years after exenteration for recurrent cervical and vulvovaginal carcinoma, found negligible reactive psychiatric morbidity, a major loss of sexual function, a substantial impact on occupational recovery and some reduction in social activity. Nonetheless, when asked, all patients affirmed that, given the chance to choose again, they would opt for exenteration, ten because the alternative was death and nine because they felt much better than prior to surgery. Overall, a significant improvement in life was reported, and each patient articulated a sense of optimism about the future.

Conclusion

Exenterative surgery, while indicated in only a small minority of patients with extensive rectal carcinoma, clearly offers the possibility of cure when all lesser procedures would leave affected patients at overwhelming risk of tumor relapse and cancer death. When performed in properly selected patients, exenteration also effectively abrogates the intractable, disabling symptoms of extensive rectal adenocarcinoma. However, these benefits are realized only at high cost in terms of operative mortality, early and late perioperative morbidity, loss of urinary, bowel, and sexual function, and major psychological adjustment. Patient selection and informed consent are therefore crucial to therapeutic success with these operations. These caveats notwithstanding, survivors report that post-exenteration quality of life is satisfactory, certainly as compared to the alternative of unrelieved symptoms and cancer mortality.

Indications for exenteration with palliative intent must be stringent. Given the recent advances in pain management and nonsurgical palliative therapy for cancer, there are few patients with incurable rectal carcinoma in whom such a radical undertaking is appropriate.

References

Boey J, Wong J, Ong GB (1982) Pelvic exenteration for locally advanced colorectal carcinoma. Ann Surg 195:513-518
Brophy PF, Hoffman JP, Eisenberg BL (1994) The role of palliative pelvic exenteration. Am J Surg 167:386-390
Deckers PJ, Olsson C, Williams LA et al (1976) Pelvic exenteration as palliation of malignant disease. Am J Surg 131:509-515
Eckhauser FE, Lindenauer SM, Morley GW (1979) Pelvic exenteration for advanced rectal carcinoma. Am J Surg 138:411-414
Falk RE, Moffat EL, Makowka L et al (1985) Pelvic exenteration for advanced primary and recurrent adenocarcinoma. Can J Surg 28:539-541
Gall FP, Tonak J, Altendorf A (1987) Multivisceral resections in colorectal cancer. Dis Colon Rectum 30:337-341
Hafner GH, Herrera L, Petrelli NJ (1991) Patterns of recurrence after pelvic exenteration for colorectal adenocarcinoma. Arch Surg 126:1510-1513
Hafner GH, Herrera L, Petrelli NJ (1992) Morbidity and mortality after pelvic exenteration for colorectal adenocarcinoma. Ann Surg 215:63-67
Hunter JA, Ryan JA, Schultz P (1987) En bloc resection of colon cancer adherent to other organs. Am J Surg 154:67-71
Jakowatz JG, Porudominsky D, Riihimaki DU et al (1985) Complications of pelvic exenteration. Arch Surg 120:1261-1265
Ketcham AS, Deckers PJ, Sugarbaker EV et al (1970) Pelvic exenteration for carcinoma of the uterine cervix. Cancer 26:513-521
Kiselow M, Butcher HR, Bricker EM (1967) Results of radical surgical treatment of advanced pelvic cancer: a fifteen year study. Ann Surg 166:428-436
Ledesma EJ, Bruno S, Mittelman A (1981) Total pelvic exenteration in colorectal carcinoma. Ann Surg 194:701-703
Lindsey WF, Wood DK, Briele HA, et al (1985) Pelvic exenteration. J Surg Oncol 30:231-234
Liu SY, Wang YN, Zhu WQ, Gu WL, Fu H (1994) Total pelvic exenteration for locally advanced rectal carcinoma. Dis Colon Rectum 37:172-174
Lopez MJ, Kraybill WG, Downey RS, Johnston WD, Bricker EM (1987) Exenterative surgery for locally advanced rectosigmoid cancers. Is it worthwhile? Surgery 102:644-651
McGlone TP, Bernie WA, Elliott DW (1982) Survival following extended operations for extracolonic invasion by colon cancer. Arch Surg 117:595-599
Moffat FL, Vargas-Cuba RD, Serafini AN et al (1994a) Radioimmunodetection of colorectal carcinoma using technetium-99m-labeled Fab' fragments of the IMMU-4 anticarcinoembyonic antigen monoclonal antibody. Cancer 73:836-845
Moffat FL, Yeung RS, Falk RE, Ketcham AS (1994b) Exenterative surgery for recurrent pelvic neoplasia. Surg Oncol Clin North Am 3:277-290
Olsson C, Deckers PJ, Williams L et al (1976) New look at pelvic exenteration. Urology 7:355-361
Pearlman NW (1994) Complications of pelvic exenteration. Surg Oncol Clin North Am 3:347-356
Pearlman NW, Donohue RE, Stiegmann GV et al (1987) Pelvic and sacropelvic exenteration for locally advanced or recurrent anorectal cancer. Arch Surg 122:537-541
Pearlman NW, Donohue RE, Wettlaufer JN et al (1990) Continent ileocolonic urinary reservoirs for filling and lining the post-exenterative pelvis. Am J Surg 160:634-637

Takagi H, Morimoto T, Yasue M, Kato K, Yamada E, Suzuki R (1985) Total pelvic exenteration for advanced carcinoma of the lower colon. J Surg Oncol 28:59-62

Temple WJ, Ketcham AS (1992) Sacral resection for control of pelvic tumors. Am J Surg 163:370-374

Vera MI (1981) Quality of life following pelvic exenteration. Gynecol Oncol 12:355-366

Wanebo HJ, Koness RJ, Turk PS, Cohen SI (1992) Composite resection of posterior pelvic malignancy. Ann Surg 215:685-695

Wanebo HJ, Koness J, Vezeridis MP, Cohen SI, Wrobleski DE (1994) Pelvic resection of recurrent rectal cancer. Ann Surg 220:586-597

Williams LF, Huddleston CB, Sawyers JL, Potts JR, Sharp KW, McDougal SW (1988) Is total pelvic exenteration reasonable primary treatment for rectal carcinoma? Ann Surg 207:670-678

Yeung RS, Moffat FL, Falk RE (1993) Pelvic exenteration for recurrent and extensive primary colorectal adenocarcinoma. Cancer 72:1853-1858

Yeung RS, Moffat FL, Falk RE (1994) Pelvic exenteration for recurrent colorectal carcinoma: a review. Cancer Invest 12:176-188

Sphincter Preservation and Sphincter Reconstruction

Coloanal J-Pouch Reconstruction Following Low Rectal Resection

K.-H. Fuchs, M. Sailer, M. Kraemer and A. Thiede

Department of Surgery, University of Würzburg,
Josef-Schneider-Strasse 2, 97080 Würzburg, Germany

Abstract

From an oncological point of view, a distal resection border of 2 cm is sufficient after deep anterior rectal resection and total mesorectal excision. This conclusion has led to extending the indications for ultradeep rectal resection in recent years. The classical end-to-end coloanal anastomosis, however, has been shown to be associated with several functional drawbacks, for example, increased stool urgency and in some cases incontinence, especially in the first 6-12 months after the operation. It was to improve these aspects that the coloanal pouch was introduced.

In a pilot study we performed a coloanal pouch in 25 patients (median age 65 years, range 32-85). The coloanal pouch anastomosis was generally performed by a stapling device. A transanal hand-sewn anastomosis was performed in the section down to the sphincter level. Indications included rectal cancer, recurrent villous adenoma, and in one case recto-vaginal fistula. The pouch was also constructed by a linear stapling device, and its length was usually 5-7 cm. The level of the anastomosis averaged 2 cm above the dentate line. In 16 patients a protective ileostomy was also carried out. We observed four cases of anastomotic leak and in one an abscess. Results showed full continence after 6 months and in 85% after 1 year. Urgency was observed in four patients after 3 months, and in only one after 1 year. In summary, we obtained encouraging results for initiating a randomized trial in the future to confirm the advantages of this type of reconstruction after deep anterior rectal resection.

Introduction

In the past 10 years sphincter-preserving techniques have been gradually accepted in the surgical therapy of rectal cancer (Parks and Percy 1982; Enker et al. 1985; Berger et al. 1992). Abdominoperineal rectal excision has become a rare approach chosen only in special circumstances (Köckerling and Gall 1994; Schumpelik and Braun 1996). The justification of this is based on published evidence that the distal resection margins in lower rectal cancer can be reduced in the vast majority of cases and the oncologic requirements for radical curative surgical therapy still be respected and fulfilled (Parks and Percy 1982; Karanjia et al. 1990; Stelzner 1989). Karanjia has shown no difference in survival between patients who underwent abdominoperineal excision and those who underwent sphincter-preserving resection (Karanjia et al. 1990).

Although patients are grateful for preservation of their natural sphincter system, their quality of life can be impaired by troublesome side-effects after the sphincter-preserving operation, such as frequent stools and stool urgency (Lazorthes et al. 1986; Karanjia et al. 1992; Hildebrandt et al. 1993). Incontinence is usually a problem in the first weeks after surgery, but continence usually is regained at the latest after several weeks. The loss of the rectal ampulla as a stool reservoir facilitating storage and infrequent, sequentially planned evacuation may be responsible for the above-mentioned problems. Possible advantages of the reconstructed rectal reservoir are of a technical and functional nature. Lazorthes introduced the J-shaped colonic pouch in 1986 (Lazorthes et al. 1986). Since then, a number of authors have gained experience with this reconstruction technique in the treatment of low rectal cancer (Parc et al. 1986; Nicholls et al. 1988; Huguet et al. 1990; Berger et al. 1992; Thiede 1993; Gross and Amir-Kabirian 1994).

One technical advantage of the coloanal pouch could be an increased anastomotic safety. A comparison between patients who had a deep anterior rectal resection with a margin lower than 1 cm and others in whom the distance of the anastomosis from the anal verge was between 3.4 and 5.8 cm showed the incidence of anastomotic leakage to be exactly the same in both groups, namely 11%. Local recurrence was not significantly different either. There were four recurrences out of 110 patients in the group where the margin was more than 1 cm between the anastomosis and the sphincter system, and no recurrences in the group ($n=42$) with the margin less than 1 cm. Very recently (Karanjia et al. 1990, 1992) LASER Doppler blood flow measurement has supported the argument that side-to-end coloanal anastomoses and unperturbed blood flow probably favor improved anastomotic healing (Hallböök et al. 1996).

A second possible advantage of the colonic reservoir is an improved functional result. Removing the lower rectum creates a temporary incontinence which usually disappears after 6–12 months, but stool frequency is still increased to up to ten stools per day. The most devastating functional problem is having a stool consistence that is quite fluid or semisolid, requiring frequent small bowel movements with an urgency that is distressing to the patient and restricts social activities. The construction of a colonic reservoir at the lower rectal location has the potential to improve these problems (Parc et al. 1986; Berger et al. 1992; Thiede 1993; Gross and Amir-Kabirian 1994; Hallböök et al. 1995; Ortiz et al. 1995).

Indications

Patient selection for lower resection rather than rectal excision must be based on a the preoperative staging and diagnostic work-up (Thiede 1993; Hildebrandt et al. 1994; Köckerling and Gall 1994; Schumpelick and Braun 1996). This must include endoscopic examination in order to determine the lower margin of the tumor with reference to the dentate line and the anal verge. In addition, possible tumor penetration of the rectal wall must be evaluated by endosonography (ES). Tumors in the lower third of the rectum should be classified into ES T1, ES T2, and those T3 tumors that merely infiltrate the rectal wall by 1-3 mm (ES T3a). In these cases, low rectal resection is indicated if the resection margin is at least 1 cm for T1 and T2 tumors or 3 cm for T3a tumors. Using the intersphincteric resection technique broadens the indication for sphincter-preserving resection even further. In all cases of T3 tumor in the middle third of the rectum, keeping sufficient resection margin and the required mesorectal excision will force the surgeon to take the resection line down to the upper end of the sphincter system. In patients with a distal rectal stump of 4-5 cm from the anal verge or even less, and patients with intersphincteric resection with sufficient anoderm on the remaining sphincter, reconstruction of the storage function above the sphincter by a J-shaped colon pouch is useful.

Technique

Since the oncologic requirements have the highest priority in these patients, the first step of the operation is isolation of the tumor by ligating the lumen of the colon at the sigmoid and then interrupting the blood flow by ligation of the inferior mesenteric vein below the pancreas and the inferior mesenteric artery near its aortic origin. Following this, the left colonic flexure is totally mobilized in order to gain sufficient length of colon to create the pouch and be able to pull it down into the pelvis without tension. The autonomous nerve bundles arc carefully dissected and left in place to prevent damage. Then the dissection is carried on down the lateral connections of the rectum, usually using sharp dissection and coagulation. The ventral and dorsal preparation proceeds stepwise until the rectum is fully mobilized from the pelvic floor. If an intersphincteric dissection is needed, it is carried out at this point.

If the tumor location allows preservation of a rectal stump, a linear stapler can be used to close the rectum distally. First the rectum should be clamped below the tumor and then an antiseptic and cytotoxic agent should be used to rinse out the rectal stump.

A second approach is the open one. Using a rectal pusher, the pelvic floor can be elevated so that the surgeon has good exposure of the rectal stump, facilitating resection of the rectum under direct vision. A purse-string suture is placed manually at the distal rectal stump (Thiede 1993). The colon anastomosis can then be completed with a circular stapler.

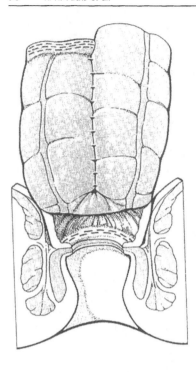

Fig. 1. Coloanal J-shaped pouch showing the coloanal anastomosis performed by a circular stapling device

A third variety of the technique is used when the tumor is located very close to the dentate line and the lowest possible safety margin with intersphincteric dissection has to be used. The index finger can be used to push away the mucosa and feel the best dividing line for resection of the rectum. The resection line will divide the rectal wall in the area of the dentate line. In this case, anastomoses with the colon pouch or the straight colon are performed transanally using manual suturing.

With the double stapling technique, a circular stapling device is used with a central pin to penetrate the linear stapling line and finally connect the rectal stump with the J-shaped colonic pouch. The latter must be prepared with the anvil of the circular stapler before connecting.

For reconstruction the descending and transverse colon are mobilized so that the descending colon can be easily moved towards the symphysis. Additional dissection of the mesentery with careful preservation of the arcades of the colon needed for blood supply may be necessary for full mobilization. The most distal 7 cm of the colon are then flipped around to double the colon (Fig. 1). Again, two possible techniques can be applied to create the pouch. One is to open the bowel at the distal end of the J-shaped colon and insert a GIA 90 from this point, the other is to open the J-shaped colon from cranially, advancing the GIA 90 down the whole length of the pouch and then penetrating the colon at the distal end of the pouch. By this technique the whole pouch can be created in one step and the cranial opening of the pouch is then closed by hand suture. As mentioned above, the distal end of

Table 1. Incidence of fistulas and abscesses with and without coloanal pouch

Series	No. of patients	Incidence of fistulas & abscesses (%)
Without pouch		
Parks and Percy 1982	76	15.6
Enker et al. 1985	41	12.2
Nicholls et al. 1988	28	21.4
Eigler and Gross 1989	70	13.4
With pouch		
Huguet et al. 1990	27	3.7
Berger et al. 1992	162	4.9
Gross and Amir-Kabirian 1994	32	3.1
Present authors' series 1995	33	15.2

Table 2. Postoperative continence with J-pouch

Series	No. of patients	Follow-up (months)	Stool frequency (per day)	Complete continence (%)	Minor troubles (%)	Fecal incontinence (%)
Lazorthes et al. 1986	42	12	1.4	43	50	7
Parc et al. 1986	136	36	1–2	52	44	4
Nicholls et al. 1988	15	47	1.4	60		
Berger et al. 1992	162	>12	1.6	88	–	<5
Wexner 1995	20	12	1.6	90	–	5

the pouch is used for direct suture with the anoderm and the sphincter at the dentate line, or the anvil of the circular stapler is introduced after placement of a circular purse-string suture to connect the pouch with the anally introduced circular stapling device. It must be emphasized that manipulating or sewing at the rectal stump from inside is always easier using a rectal pusher from the anal route. When we were first beginning to use this technique, we always combined the coloanal pouch with a temporary ileostomy for safety reasons (Thiede 1993).

Results and Comment

Table 1 shows the results of published studies summarized as to the incidence of fistulas and abscesses after rectal excision and reconstruction with and without coloanal pouches. The data demonstrate clearly that there is a trend to reduced fistulas and abscesses in patients in whom a pouch has been used to perform the coloanal anastomosis. This has also been verified by the two randomized trials that have been completed so far (Hallböök et

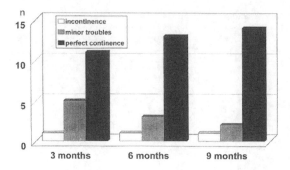

Fig. 2. Development of postoperative continence after J-pouch reconstruction ($n=16$). At 3 months patients already have acceptable continence with improvement at 9 months

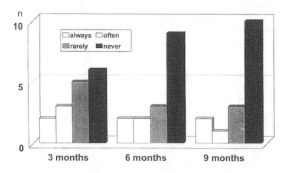

Fig. 3. Development of stool urgency after J-pouch reconstruction ($n=16$). Only 50% of patients suffer from urgency 3 months after the operation. By 9 months it is improved in most patients

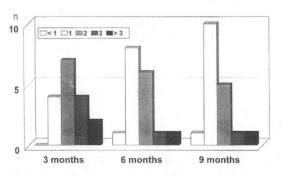

Fig. 4. Postoperative stool frequency after J-pouch: Only a minority of patients pass more than 3 stools per day after 9 months postoperatively

al. 1995; Seow-Choen et al. 1995). Both studies also show functional advantages. Table 2 shows data from studies of postoperative continence. On the basis of these data, at least half of the patients can be regarded as completely continent after the operation; complete fecal incontinence occurs in less than 5%–7%. An important finding after colonic pouch formation is the improvement in stool frequency, shown in Table 2. Randomized trials have also shown this advantage for the patients in the group with coloanal pouches (Hallböök et al. 1995; Seow-Choen et al. 1995).

Results from our own pilot study are illustrated in Figs. 2–4. These figures show the postoperative course of patients after J-pouch reconstruction with regard to stool frequency, urgency, and postoperative continence. The data clearly show, as did other studies, that stool frequency after J-pouch reconstruction is reduced to an average number of 1-2 stools per day and the incidence of quality-of-life-reducing urgency is present in only a minority of the patients (Figs. 3, 4).

On the basis of recently published results, reconstruction with a J-shaped coloanal pouch after lower rectal dissection seems to have several advantages over straight anastomosis. Major advantages are possibly improved anastomotic safety, a lower incidence of fistulas and abscesses, and, especially, long-term postoperative functional improvements for the patients. Regarding the functional criteria, an interesting finding is reduced stool frequency and a reduced incidence of urgency in the patients. It is therefore most important to evaluate this trend in more randomized clinical trials with long-term oncologic and functional follow-up, so that if appropriate the procedure can become standard in the near future.

References

Berger A, Tiret E, Parc R et al (1992) Excision of the rectum with colonic J pouch - anal anastomosis for adenocarcinoma of the low and mid rectum. World J Surg 16:470-477

Eigler FW, Gross E (1989) Die peranale Anastomose nach Rektumresektion. Langenbecks Arch Klin Chir Suppl 794

Enker WE, Stearns MW, Janov AJ (1985) Peranal coloanal anastomosis following low anterior resection for rectal carcinoma. Dis Colon Rectum 28:576-581

Gross E, Amir-Kabirian H (1994) Koloanaler Pouch nach totaler Rektumresektion. Zentralbl Chir 119:878-885

Hallböök O, Påhlman L, Krog M, Wexner SD, Sjödahl R (1995) Prospective randomized comparison between straight and colonic J-pouch anastomosis after low anterior resection (abstract). Dis Colon Rectum 38:P21

Hallböök O, Johansson K, Sjödahl R (1996) Laser Doppler blood flow measurement in rectal resection for carcinoma - comparison between the straight and colonic J pouch reconstruction. Br J Surg 83:389-392

Hildebrandt U, Zuther T, Lindemann W, Ecker K (1993) Elektromyographische Funktion des coloanalen Pouches. Langenbecks Areh Chir 127-131

Hildebrandt U, et al (1994) Der koloanale Pouch: Indikation, Funktion und Ergebnisse. Zentralbl Chir 119: 886-891

Huguet C, Harb J, Bona S (1990) Coloanal anastomosis after resection of low rectal cancer in the elderly. World J Surg 14:619-623

Karanjia ND, Schache DJ, North WRS, Heald RJ (1990) "Close shave" in anterior resection. Br J Surg 77:510-512

Karanjia ND, Schache DJ, Heald RJ (1992) Function of the distal rectum after low anterior resection for carcinoma. Br J Surg 79:114-116

Köckerling F, Gall FP (1994) Chirurgische Standards beim Rektumkarzinom. Chirurg 65:593-603

Lazorthes F, Fages P, Chiotasso P, Lemozy J, Bloom E (1986) Resection of the rectum with construction of a colonic reservoir and coloanal anastomosis for carcinoma of the rectum. Br J Surg 73:136-138

Nicholls RJ, Lubouski DZ, Donaldson DR (1988) Comparison of colonic reservoir and straight colo-anal reconstruction after rectal excision. Br J Surg 75:318-320

Ortiz H, De Miguel M, Armendáriz P, et al (1995) Coloanal anastomosis: are functional results better with a pouch? Dis Colon Rectum 38:375-377

Parc R, Tiret E, Frileux P, Moszkowski E, Loynge J (1986) Resection and colo-anal anastomosis with colonic reservoir for rectal carcinoma. Br J Surg 73:139-141
Parks AG, Percy JP (1982) Resection and sutured colo-anal anastomosis for rectal carcinoma. Br J Surg 69:301-304
Schumpelick V, Braun J (1996) Die intersphinktäre Rektumresektion mit radikaler Mesorektumexzision und coloanaler Anastomose. Chirurg 67:110-120
Seow-Choen F, Goh HS (1995) Prospective randomized trial comparing J colonic pouch - anal anastomosis and straight coloanal reconstruction. Br J Surg 82:608-610
Stelzner F (1989) Die Begründung, die Technik und die Ergebnisse der knappen Kontinenzresektion. Langenbecks Arch Chir Suppl II 675
Thiede A (1993) Kolorektaler, koloanaler Pouch. In: Fuchs K-H, Engemann R, Thiede A (eds) Klammernahttechnik in der Chirurgie. Springer, Berlin Heidelberg New York, pp 144-150

Seromuscular Spiral Cuff Perineal Colostomy: An Alternative to Abdominal Wall Colostomy After Abdominoperineal Excision for Rectal Cancer

P. M. Schlag, W. Slisow, and K. T. Moesta

Department of Surgery and Surgical Oncology, Robert Rössle Hospital, Charité Humboldt University of Berlin, Lindenberger Weg 80, 13122 Berlin, Germany

Abstract

Seromuscular spiral cuff perineal colostomy may be an alternative to abdominal wall colostomy after abdomino-perineal excision. We present our initial experience with the procedure in 13 patients operated upon between March 1993 and December 1997. Patients undergoing abdomino-perineal excision for rectal cancer, under 65 years of age, without severe concomitant disease, and strongly motivated to comply with an intensive postoperative physiotherapy were selected. The neosphincter procedure comprised a pull-through of a sufficient length of well-vascularized colon, 12 cm of which was then cleared of fat. In this segment, the seromuscular layer was separated from the mucosa, cut into a longitudinal sheet and wrapped in spirals around the colon at its perineal insertion. One patient died from pulmonary embolism. A second patient suffered from ischemic necrosis of the distal colon and lost his neosphincter. Minor complications included one stenosis, corrected by surgery, and one iatrogenic lesion on rectoscopy at another institution. No patients experienced local recurrence, while four patients presented distant metastases. Initially, all patients suffered from incontinence. After 6 months, 6 of 11 evaluable patients showed total and 5 showed partial continence.

Introduction

Although handling procedures and patient aids for abdominal wall colostomies have substantially improved with time, the concurrent psychological trauma and social restrictions are still severe. The reduction in life quality of course depends on the individual's social activities and esthetic demands (Cohen 1991). A perineal colostomy would in principle prevent the disfigurement, however, it hampered by substantial handling problems. A method described for the first time in 1989 by Fedorov et al. may enable the development of such perineal colostomy imitating the inner sphincter by a spiral apposition of multiple seromuscular layers from the large bowel (Fedorov et al. 1986). We present our initial surgical experience with this technique.

Table 1. Characteristics and functional results of 13 patients undergoing the seromuscular spiral cuff perineal colostomy procedure

No.	Age (years)	Sex	Tumor stage	Pretreatment	Function	Continence score[a]
1	56	M	yrpT3N0G2	RT	Sufficient	12
2	67	M	pT2N0G1		–	–
3	66	F	pT3N1G2		Sufficient	9
4	50	M	pT3N3G2		Good	16
5	55	F	pT2N0G2		Good	15
6	60	M	ypT2N1G2	HRCT	Good	13
7	66	M	ypT0NTG2	HRCT	Good	14
8	59	M	pT2N1G2		Sufficient	12
9	45	F	pT3N1G2		–	–
10	56	F	ypT3N2G3	HRCT	Good	15
11	65	M	ypT3N0G2	HRCT	Sufficient	12
12	58	M	ypT3N0G2	HRCT	Good	13
13	64	M	ypT2N0G2	HRCT	Sufficient	12

RT, External radiotherapy; HRCT, hyperthermic radiochemotherapy. functional results: good, continent for liquids and stool, some incontinence for gas; sufficient, continent for stool, some incontinence for liquids.
[a] According to Herold and Bruch (1996)

Patients and Methods

Patients

Between March 1993 and December 1997 we performed primary seromuscular spiral cuff perineal colostomies during abdomino-perineal excision in 13 patients with rectal cancer. Patient characteristics are presented in Table 1. These 13 account for 21% of a total of 62 patients treated during this period with rectal cancer in similar location, within 3–6 cm of the anocutaneous line, and T2 or T3 tumor infiltration of the bowel wall. Patients aged under 65 years, strongly motivated, able and willing to proceed with an intensive postoperative physiotherapy were selected for the seromuscular neosphincter perineal colostomy. Multiple colonic diverticula and severe concomitant disease were exclusion criteria. One patient had preoperative external radiotherapy (40 Gy). Six patients had preoperative hyperthermic radiochemotherapy (five cycles of microwave hyperthermia, 5-fluorouracil, leucovorin, and 42 Gy external radiation) with four postoperative cycles of systemic chemotherapy (5-fluorouracil and leucovorin) for locally advanced (uT3 and uT4) or recurrent ($n=1$) disease.

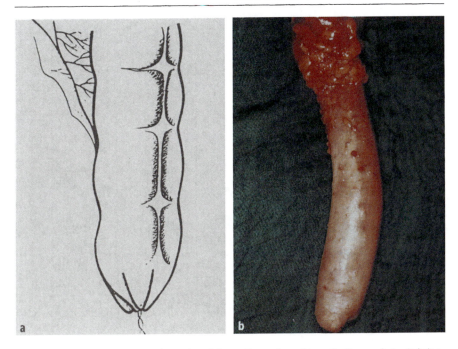

Fig. 1a,b. The distal end of the colon is cleared from adjacent fat. **a** Schematic diagram. **b** Surgical situation

Surgical Procedure and Postoperative Care

The abdominoperineal excision was performed in accordance with standard oncological criteria, with no compromise as to radicality in view of the sphincter neoformation to follow. Our standard includes total mesorectal excision, removal of the entire external and internal sphincter apparatus, and lymphatic dissection up to the root of the centrally ligated inferior mesenteric artery. After the resection was completed, in general by a two-team approach, the colon was transsected at the descendosigmoidal junction. The specimen was removed through the perineum. The remainders of the levatoric muscles and of the anococcygeal ligament were then identified and labeled by sutures. In the abdominal cavity the descending part of the colon, the left flexure, and the transverse colon were mobilized and separated from the major omentum, respecting the pericolic arcade and preserving the vascular supply from the middle colonic artery. For the spiral seromuscular cuff formation, first the distal end of the colon over a distance of 12 cm was freed from pericolic fat (Fig. 1).

A subtile and time-consuming preparation separated the seromuscular layer from the colonic mucosa (Fig. 2). Care had to be taken not to perforate the mucosal tube so as to avoid contamination and peristomal infection. The resulting 10- to 12-cm-long seromuscular tube was then cut in a spiral way

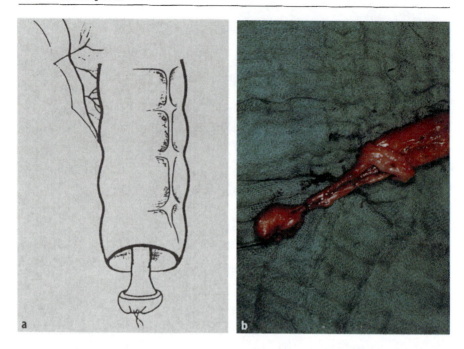

Fig. 2a, b. The mucosa is carefully separated from the seromuscular tube. **a** Schematic diagram. **b** Surgical situation

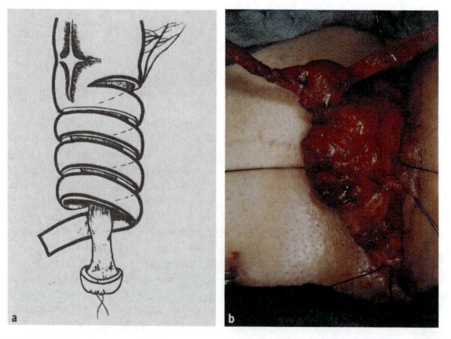

Fig. 3a, b. A seromuscular sheet is formed from the tube by spiral incision. **a** Schematic diagram. **b** Surgical situation

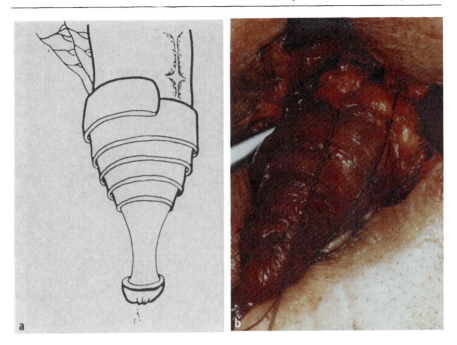

Fig. 4a, b. The cuff is formed by spiral apposition of the seromuscular sheet. **a** Schematic diagram. **b** Surgical situation

to form a longitudinal sheet 25 cm long and 2.5 cm wide, still attached at its base to the vascularized colonic wall (Fig. 3). This seromuscular sheet was wrapped around the distal end of the intact colon, while each spiral tour was sutured to the intact serosa (Fig. 4). The sheet was carefully prestretched both in length and width prior to the wrapping (Schmidt and Peiper 1972). The resulting seromuscular cuff was approximately 5 cm long; the opening of the cuff had to allow elastic passage of an index finger (28–30 charriere). The colon wearing the seromuscular cuff was then pulled through into the perineal opening (Fig. 5).

Closing the perineum layer by layer, care was taken to fix the labeled remainders of levator muscles and anococcygeal ligament to the colonic serosa above the cuff in order to form a stoma slightly retracted from the skin level and to reconstruct a somewhat physiological angle of the distal colon within the perineum. A deviation colostomy was necessary in a single patient who received an additional colonic pouch procedure. In this case the colostomy was closed 3 months later. The perineal cavity was drained for 3–5 days. All patients were covered by antibiotics (ceftriaxon and metronidazole) for 5 days. Some 10–12 days after surgery an intensive physiotherapy of the pelvic, gluteal, and thigh musculature was initiated aimed at compensating for the lack of external sphincter. This special training program was continued for 3–6 months. To stabilize the cuff tension an intermittent electrostimula-

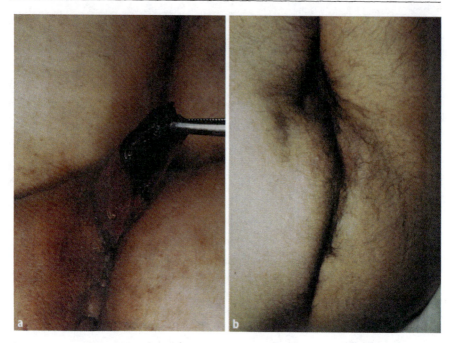

Fig. 5. a Perineal colostomy. On day 5 the remainder of mucosal tube exceeding the stoma is necrotic; the stoma itself is well vascularized (patient no. 10). **b** Perineal colostomy 3 months after surgery. The slightly funnel-like situation hides the colostomy between the gluteal muscles (patient no. 4)

tion was applied by a point electrode in contact with the perineal colostomy. The sphincter training was further enhanced by a biofeedback procedure, which was also carried out for 3–6 months. Patients were usually dismissed from the hospital after 3 weeks. Continence scores were evaluated based on the work of Herold and Bruch (1996).

Results

Postoperative Complications

One diabetic patient (patient no. 2) suffered ischemic necrosis of the distal colon including the neosphincter. He underwent a second laparotomy, partial colonic resection, and definitive abdominal wall colostomy. A second, obese patient (no. 9) died from fulminant pulmonary embolism on the 12th day after surgery; autopsy revealed a regular postoperative site, the embolism originating from pelvic vein thrombosis. Ten patients experienced no postoperative morbidity.

The first patient operated upon (no. 1) developed a stricture of his colostomy 4 months after the initial operation, which was subject to surgical correction by superficial excision of the contracted scar and reimplantation of the colostomy. In a second patient (no. 7) a rigid rectoscopy was attempted at an outside hospital 2 months after surgery. He suffered a perforation of the colon and a partial disruption of the perineal stoma. Initial healing was observed after deviation colostomy; however, a peristomal prolapse had to be corrected by a complete renewal of the perineal seromuscular sphincter procedure with concomitant closure of the deviation colostomy.

Oncological Results

No patient experienced a locoregional recurrence (median follow-up 25 months, range 8-57 months). Four patients suffered distant metastases. One of these (no. 3) died 22 months after surgery from multiple liver metastases. The second (no. 8) had a solitary liver metastasis resected 23 months after the initial operation; he has remained free of recurrence for 12 months. The third (no. 10) experienced supraclavicular lymph node metastases 9 months after surgery and is currently being treated by combination chemotherapy. Patient no. 12 suffers from pulmonary metastases and is being treated by systemic chemotherapy.

Functional Results

Initially all patients suffered from incontinence. Bowel movements were arrhythmic and occurred 8-15 times per day. Necessity was not perceived during the first 30 days. Thereafter the patients learned to counteract a necessity for 1-5 min. Slowly they developed the ability to discriminate between solid or liquid stool and gas. The frequency of bowel movements declined to 1-3 per day. The duration of bowel emptying was eventually prolonged and fragmented within 20-60 min. The resulting continence scores 6 months after surgery are represented in Table 1. Six patients showed "total" and five partial continence. One patient (no. 1) uses irrigation to improve upon safety during his frequent business travels.

Discussion

Abdominoperineal excision remains the method of choice for the majority of cancers of the lower third of the rectum, except those of very early stage amenable to local excision. The concomitant necessity of a permanent abdominal wall colostomy with uncontrolled bowel emptying reduces the patient's quality of life in physical, mental, and social ways (Cohen 1991). In the past numerous attempts have been made to imitate the complex sphincteric system at least partially in order to compensate the negative functional effects of the abdominoperineal excision (Abercrombie and Williams 1995). The most intensive research so far has focused on neosphincter procedures using skeletal muscle. However, the procedures initially proposed for treating incontinence showed little benefit when applied after abdominoperineal excision. This is due mainly to the skeletal muscles' (type II fibers) inability for long-lasting contraction. The finding that type II fibers may be transformed into type I fibres able to contract continuously by stimulation with low-frequency currents led to the development of a double-sided transposition graciloplasty, submitted to continuous stimulation by an implanted pacemaker (George et al. 1993; Salmons and Henrisson 1981; Williams et al. 1990). The procedure is extensive, entails considerable morbidity, and due to the pacemaker is expensive (Geerdes et al. 1995). The use of smooth musculature, such as from the bowel wall itself, seems preferable with regard to the skeletal muscles' functional limitations. However, Schmidt et al. failed when they tried to create a continent abdominal wall colostomy by cylindrically cuffing the stomal colon with free transplants of autologous large bowel musculature (Beger et al. 1982; Schmidt et al. 1979). The majority of their patients experienced stomal strictures or peristomal abscesses. The major reason for this may have been the lack of vasculature supply to the transplant with consecutive necrosis and scar formation.

The seromuscular spiral cuff technique preserves the microvasculature of the cuff, as demonstrated by extensive animal studies [2]. The spiral apposition with moderate overlap of the thin sheet against the well-vascularized pericolic tissue may add to the oxygenation of the graft by diffusion. Except for iatrogenic colon perforation, only one patient suffered a severe, procedure-related complication. He experienced necrosis of the distal colon, including the cuff, which was due to still insufficient mobilization of the colon. This patient was the fourth one operated on, and similar problems can be avoided with growing experience. Although some of the patients were pretreated by radiochemotherapy, no perineal wound healing problems occurred, and adjuvant therapy was never delayed due to the neosphincter procedure. However, the hospital stay was deliberately longer, due to the novelty of the procedure, the initial incontinence, and the intensive training program. As far as such a conclusion can be drawn at all based on a small number of patients, no survival deficit was observed among the patients treated with inclusion of the neosphincter procedure compared to stage-matched historical controls.

Thus we are able to confirm the findings of Fedorov et al. (1986; Odaryuk 1995) with regard to an acceptable level of pseudocontinence obtained in the majority of patients.

References

Abercrombie JE, Williams NS (1995) Total anorectal reconstruction. Br J Surg 82:438
Beger HG, Schmidt E, Pistor G (1982) Die Rekonstruktion des Anus naturalis durch Transplantation glatter Darmmuskulatur. Chirurg 53:599
Cohen A (1991) Body image change in the person with a stoma. J Enterostoma 18:68

Fedorov VD, Odaryuk TS, Shelygin YA, et al (1986) Method of creation of a smooth-muscle cuff at the site of the perineal colostomy after extirpation of the rectum. Dis Colon Rectum 32:562

Geerdes BP, Zoetmulder FAN, Baeten CGMI (1995) Double dynamic graciloplasty and coloperineal pull-through after abdomino-perineal resection. Eur J Cancer 31A:1248

George BD, Williams NS, Patel J, et al (1993) Physiological and histochemical adaptation of the electrically stimulated gracillis muscle to neoanal sphincter function. Br J Surg 80:1342

Herold A, Bruch HP (1996) Stufendiagnostik der anorektalen Inkontinenz. Zentralbl Chir 121:320

Odaryuk TS (1995) Personal communication

Salmons S, Henrisson J (1981) The adaptive response of skeletal muscle to increased use. Muscle Nerve 4:94

Schmidt E, Peiper U (1972) The importance of the initial stretch for activation of the isolated vascular smooth muscle. Pflugers Arch 332:75

Schmidt E, Bruch HP, Greulich M, et al (1979) Kontinente Kolostomie durch freie Transplantation autologer Dickdarmmuskulatur. Chirurg 50:96

Williams NS, Hallan RJ, Koeze TI, et al (1990) Restoration of gastrointestinal continuity and continence after abdomino-perineal excision of the rectum using an electrically stimulated neoanal sphincter. Dis Colon Rectum 33:561

Total Anorectal Reconstruction Supported by Electrostimulated Gracilis Neosphincter

E. Cavina, M. Seccia, and M. Chiarugi

Department of Surgery, University of Pisa, S. Chiara Hospital, via Roma 67, 56124 Pisa, Italy

Abstract

Purpose: To review and to update the results of Total Anorectal Reconstruction with Electrostimulated Graciloplasty (ES-TAR) at the same time as or following abdominoperineal resection (APR). *Setting:* A university hospital in Italy. *Methods:* Retrospective study. *Population:* A series of 98 consecutive anorectal cancer patients who had undergone ES-TAR (in 88 cases at the same time as APR; in 10 cases following APR), 61 of whom are still evaluable in respect of continence (median follow-up period 55 months). *Results:* There was no mortality. Thirty-seven percent of patients had postoperative complications with no impact on survival or functional outcome. The 5-year survival rate in 50 patients was 61% and the 5-year estimated cumulative probability of survival in 81 patients was 65%. Local recurrence rate was 16%. Continence was achieved in 87% of patients with a chronically stimulated TAR, and in 69% of patients with short-term stimulation. *Conclusion:* ES-TAR is a safe and effective method for both curing anorectal cancer and restoring continence. It may be considered a reliable alternative to sphincter-saving procedures in lower rectal cancer patients.

Introduction

Abdominoperineal resection (APR) to cure cancer of the rectum and sigmoid was first introduced by E.H. Miles in 1908 (Miles 1908), and since then reducing the need for a permanent colostomy has become a major and ambitious objective of colorectal surgeons. Among the methods adopted to attain this purpose, total anorectal reconstruction (TAR) after APR is the most recent. This newly introduced term (Williams 1992; Abercrombie and Williams 1995; Roseau 1995) applies to a surgical procedure that follows anorectal extirpation and is based on the construction of a perineal colostomy with a new sphincteric system consisting of either a standard or an electrically stimulated graciloplasty. The construction of the myoplasty may also employ the abductor muscle, muscular flaps from the glutei, or smooth muscle according to Schmidt's procedure.

Electromyostimulation (EMS) activates the new sphincter by contracting muscular fibers to obtain continence (Cavina et al. 1981, 1982, 1993; Mercati et al. 1991; Geerdees et al. 1995). EMS of the new sphincteric apparatus can be variously provided; one possibility is an implantable pulse generator (IPG) (Baeten et al. 1988, 1991; Williams et al. 1990; Geerdees et al. 1995).

The EMS-supported graciloplasty (restorative perineal graciloplasty, RPG) is the reconstructive method that since 1981 (Cavina et al. 1981) we have studied and applied in the field of anorectal cancer and fecal incontinence. The architectural design of this model was developed from the idea that a functionally reliable newly constructed sphincter should reproduce as far as possible the normal anatomy of the anal sphincter, and thus should have a static (anorectal angle) and a dynamic anatomic muscular component.

We have reviewed data and results from a 15-year experience. Some of these results, following the evolution of the surgical technique, have been previously reported (Cavina 1996; Cavina et al. 1987, 1990; Seccia et al. 1994). This paper gives an overview of our clinical research and experience, and highlights the results from a group of patients operated on between 1985 and 1990, with a minimum follow-up period of 5 years.

Patients and Methods

Patient Population

During a surgical experience lasting over 10 years (January 1985 to September 1995), 98 patients underwent TAR and RPG supported by short- and/or long-term electrostimulation protocols (ES-TAR). ES-TAR was carried out in 88 patients simultaneously with an APR of the anorectum for lower rectal cancer and in 10 patients as a reconstructive procedure following previous APR.

In four patients, colonic ischaemia complications that occurred intraoperatively or during the first 12 hrs postoperatively obliged us to convert perineal colostomies in to abdominal colostomies, without further significant complications; these patients are not included in the functional study. Admission criteria and patient distribution are summarized in Table 1 and follow-up data in Table 2. From February 1986 to the present date, following preliminary experience in three patients, standardized short-term and chronic electrostimulation protocols were also adopted in 21 patients subjected to graciloplasty for end-stage faecal incontinence.

All patients subjected to ES-TAR were evaluated preoperatively and during the subsequent follow-up period according to standard oncological protocols. Neosphincteric function was periodically evaluated by the same surgical team, using continence questionnaires, scores (continence diary, modified Corman's scores, modified Williams Scale), and physical examination (static

Table 1. Distribution of patients and admission criteria

Timing of total anorectal reconstruction with electrostimulated gracioplasty	Admission criteria	Mean patient age (years)	Patient sex	No. of patients evaluable for continence
Simultaneous with abdominoperineal resection ($n=88$)	Lower rectal cancer (mean height 2.5 cm) Karnofsky Performance Scale >50 Sphincter-saving procedure not feasible No evidence of extrarectal spread	62.1	m 60 f 28	51
Following earlier abdominoperineal resection ($n=10$)	Poor quality of life Complications of abdominal colostomy Karnofsky Performance Scale >50 No evidence of tumour recurrence	56.4	m 3 f 7	10
Total ($n=98$)		61.5	m 63 f 35	61

Table 2. Follow-up and continence evaluability ($n=98$)

Early conversion to abdominal colostomy	4	Left colon ischaemia	4
Died during study	28	Cancer recurrence	24
		Others	4
Lost to follow-up	1		
Converted to abdominal colostomy for late complications or cancer recurrence	3	Pelvic recurrence	2
		Late perineal hernia	1
In training (early postoperative course)	1		
Evaluable for continence	61/98	Free from cancer	53
		With cancer recurrence	8

and dynamic electromanometry, endoscopy, endoluminal sonography and defaecography). Furthermore, in 1994, 37 patients subjected to ES-TAR between 1985 and 1991, thus having a minimum of 3 years of follow-up study, were personally checked by the first author.

At present, 61 patients are clinically evaluable for continence, with a median follow-up of 55 months. Thirty-six of these (median follow-up: 84.8 months) were subjected to short-term electrostimulation and biofeedback protocols, while the last 25 (median follow-up: 19 months) underwent chronic electrostimulation, supported by IPG.

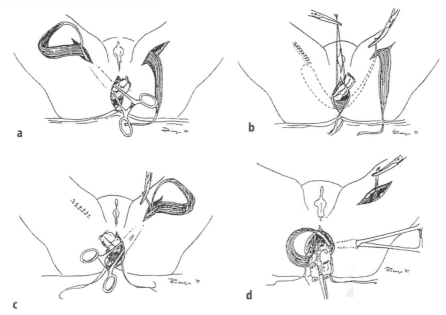

Fig. 1. a,b Mobilizing and tunnelling the gracilis sling around the colon. **c,d** Mobilizing and tunnelling the gracilis to encircle the colon

Surgical Technique and Electrostimulation

Currently, the steps of the surgical procedure are standardized as follows. It is important to have a viable proximal segment of left colon long enough to be delivered through the perineum without traction. When criteria of oncological radicality are met, the levator ani muscles should be dissected free. The levator ani insertions will provide steady anchoring points for the RPG. During the APR, the gracilis muscles are dissected free from the thighs. Special care is taken to preserve the proximal pedicle of the muscle, where the neurovascular bundle runs.

The colonic stump is delivered through the perineum for a distance of 4–5 cm. After a few days, any excess colon is resected and the perineal colostomy is mucocutaneously sutured to the perineum. Late maturing of the perineal colostomy may reduce perineal infections.

The gracilis muscles are mobilized and transposed to the perineum following Pickrell's original scheme. The left gracilis surrounds the perineal colostomy in clockwise "alpha"-shaped wrap, reproducing the anatomy and function of the external sphincter. The right gracilis is placed in a retrocolic position to simulate puborectalis sling function (dynamic and static graciloplasty) (Fig. 1 a, b).

The tendons of both gracilis muscles are fixed subcutaneously. It should be emphasized that the configuration of these muscles with respect to the stoma endows the RPG anatomically and physiologically with static and dynamic properties.

As experience was acquired and the availability of electrostimulation devices changed, various models of electrode implant were adopted. In the first series, after nerve identification with a disposable nerve locator (Pulsatron nerve stimulator, Weck, USA), steel electrodes (Temporary Pacing Wire, Ethnor SA, Neuilly, France) were placed directly on the main nerve surface of each transposed muscle, then passed through the abdominal skin for external stimulation. In the next series, where implantable devices enabled the total stimulation time to be prolonged, steel electrodes were connected by extension cables to monopolar and/or bipolar IPGs (Itrel model 7421, 7420, Medtronic, Kerkrade, The Netherlands). Finally, in the most recent experience with chronic electrostimulation (1991-1995), special platinum-iridium electrodes were connected to quadripolar IPGs (Itrel II model 7424 and SP5548 and 4300 model leads, Kerkrade, The Netherlands).

When short-term stimulation was adopted (69 patients), the duration of EMS (median 3 months; range 1-18 months) was directly influenced by electrode displacement, lead infection and patient discomfort. Short-term stimulation proved its effectiveness in preventing muscular atrophy and improving gracilis contraction strength. At the same time, the evidence of neosphincter contraction enabled patients to comply better with biofeedback protocols.

With the aim of increasing muscular resistance to continuous stimulation and prolonged contraction, chronic stimulation has been adopted in the last 27 patients subjected to ES-TAR. Quadripolar IPGs and platinum-iridium electrodes proved their safety and efficacy to guarantee long-term stimulation (median 19 months; range 1-46 months). Details of the chronic electrostimulation protocol have been published elsewhere (Cavina et al. 1987, 1990; Seccia et al. 1994).

Summary of Technique. The key points of the surgical procedure are: (a) double gracilopasty, (b) tendons fixed to soft structures, (c) both muscles anchored to levator ani stumps, (d) protective abdominal colostomy unnecessary, (e) delayed maturing of the perineal stoma, and (f) one-stage procedure for RPG and electrodes and IPG implantation.

Results

Functional Results

At present, 61 patients are fully evaluable for continence and physical investigations (median follow-up 55 months); 36 of these patients (first series) were previously subjected to short-term electrostimulation protocols and still perform muscular exercises to maintain muscular activity, and 25 receive chronic electrostimulation from implantable devices. After ES-TAR continence was achieved in 47 patients (77%). The procedure failed in 4 patients

(7%), in whom daily colonic washing was necessary, and various degrees of incontinence were observed in the remaining 10 (16%). Comparing the short-term stimulated group ($n=36$) with the chronically stimulated group ($n=25$), continence rates of 69% and 87% respectively were observed.

Oncological Results

The overall crude 5-year survival rate in 50 patients is 56%. Excluding non-cancer-related deaths, the rate is 61%. The estimated cumulative probability of survival at 5 years based on 81 patients is 65%. Local recurrence was observed in 16% of patients, who had a mean of 46.5 months disease-free. Comparison of our data to those in the literature suggests that the anorectal cancer cure rate has not been diminished by simultaneous TAR and RPG.

Discussion

The first part of the discussion concerns the "philosophy" that led to the adoption of the surgical procedure.

Since the last decade, the impressive increase in sphincter–saving procedures has reduced the number of patients requiring a permanent stoma for the cure of rectal cancer. Many reports (Graf et al. 1990; Beart et al. 1995; Enker et al. 1995) with few dissenters (Abulafi and Williams 1994), show long-term survival and disease-free interval of patients with mid- and low-rectal cancers to be mostly the same whether they are managed by low anterior resection or APR. In addition, innovative procedures have been recently adopted to preserve the anal sphincter in anal and rectal cancers diagnosed by ultrasound as low-stage and technically not amenable to resection. These include local excisional procedures and transanal endoscopic microsurgery (Buess et al. 1992; Schlag, this volume).

A recent survey of the Commission on Cancer of the American College of Surgeons (Beart et al. 1995), investigating 10 293 patients operated on for rectal cancer, indicates, however that the frequency with which APR is performed went down only slightly, from 29.3% to 25.3% for cases diagnosed between 1983 and 1988. In 1983, 7.4% of stage 0 (AJCC), 32.7% of stage I and 35.2% of stage II anorectal cancers were managed by APR, while in 1988 this was done in 6.3%, 26.1% and 30.9% of cases respectively.

These facts suggest that, despite innovations in surgery and in adjuvant therapeutics, some patients with anorectal cancer will always require APR to be cured. These patients are bound to carry a permanent abdominal stoma. Even when rectal cancer has been successfully managed by "extreme" conservative surgery and coloanal or very low colorectal anastomosis, some concerns exist about postoperative functional results. Loss of discrimination of bowel content, urge to void, tenesmus, soiling and incontinence are common drawbacks reported after rectal extirpation.

The impact of the J-colonic pouch, the surgical stratagem that has been claimed to prevent these disturbances, should be carefully evaluated. According to Paty (Paty et al. 1994), in a long-term follow-up study of 81 patients who have undergone low anterior resection and J-pouch construction, functional results remain fair in 32% of cases and poor in 12%. In the opinion of Sun et al. (1994), the crucial point for poor functional results is the after-stapler instability of the internal anal sphincter. For the same operation performed on 103 patients, Staimmer (Staimmer and Kugler 1995) reports a good functional result in 80%, with complete continence in 68% on long-term evaluation, but emphasizes that only 41% of patients achieved continence in the 1st year after surgery. In the series reported by Leo et al. (1995), 71% of patients achieved complete continence after colonic J-pouch construction, or, in other words, 29% are incompletely continent. Occasional and frequent episodes of incontinence were reported in 18% and 4% of cases respectively by Berger et al. (1992).

The lessons to be drawn from the above oncological and functional data may be summarized as follows: we can reduce (but not eliminate) the need for APR by adopting more conservative procedures, but in so doing we have to pay a steady and significant cost in term of functional disorders. Our and other authors' development of TAR and RPG techniques (Baeten et al. 1988; Mercati et al. 1991; Williams 1992; Santoro et al. 1994; Abercrombie and Williams 1995; Geerdees et al. 1995) has been based on the aim of allowing good quality of life to patients operated on for rectal cancer. Conceptually, this procedure allows a more radical (perhaps also safer?) approach to cancer, with functional results often similar to and sometimes better than those obtained by less demolitive surgery.

The second part of this discussion focuses on our clinical experience. Some crucial points to be discussed include the selection of patients, complications, quality of life after TAR and the delivery of adjuvant therapy. These points were raised as questions following the oral presentation of this paper at the Conference in Berlin.

Patient Selection

TAR is indicated in patients judged unsuited to more conservative surgery (low anterior resection, coloanal anastomosis, transanal endoscopic, microsurgery). A high risk of recurrence should be a contraindication for the procedure, on the grounds of the lack of long-life expectancy for patient and/or for his RPG. Patients should be carefully selected on the basis of preoperative staging of the tumour. Whether TAR is indicated in the elderly with non-advanced cancer is still unclear.

Complications

A high incidence of perineal complications challenges patients undergoing TAR. These complications include acute bowel ischaemia, acute prolapse, perineal infection, stoma dislocation, partial muscular necrosis, fistula, stricture and tendon impairment. Nevertheless, the occurrence of complications has declined from 41% recorded for patients operated on between 1985 and 1989 to 33% for patients operated on between 1990 and 1994.

The improvement in complication rate may be attributed to increased surgical experience. Late maturing of the perineal colostomy has also dramatically reduced the occurrence of perineal wound infection. The routine adoption of proximal diverting colostomy did not prove to be significant for reducing complications.

Once infection has developed, prompt debridement with saline irrigation of the perineal wound is the simplest and most effective method of treatment.

Quality of Life

Seventy-five percent of the patients operated on maintain the practice of a daily or every-other-day enema. For most of them this is a little enema that has the function of making voiding easier and preventing soiling. For instance, patients undergoing chronic EMS provoke daily colonic voiding by introducing 200 ml warm saline once the IPG has been switched off. No patient employs a colonic irrigation regimen to avoid faecal incontinence, as erroneously believed by some authors (Abercrombie and Williams 1995).

Twenty-five percent of operated patients experienced some degree of soiling from the newly formed anus. In most cases, mucous soiling was due to ectropion of the stomal mucosa, and it was successfully managed by anoplasty. This procedure was performed in 13 patients.

Adjuvant Therapy

Some patients received radiotherapy before or after surgery, but the lack of study protocols about irradiation, make it impossible to draw any definitive conclusions. When adjuvant therapy was given, it was not shown to have negatively influenced the dissection during surgery or the postoperative complication rate and functional outcome.

Transient episodes of incontinence may afflict patients who have undergone TAR and RPG as a side effect of postoperative adjuvant chemotherapy. Mucositis of the gastrointestinal tract may lead to poorly formed stools that may possibly not be controlled by an as yet untrained RPG. For those patients in whom postoperative adjuvant therapy is required, low-side-effect regimens of radiotherapy and chemotherapy may be desirable (Påhlman, this volume).

Conclusion

The 5-year survival rate and the postoperative complication rate associated with total anorectal reconstruction (TAR) plus restorative perineal graciloplasty are within the range reported in the literature for standard abdominoperineal resection. Long-term follow-up shows that TAR supported by short-term electromyostimulation is effective in both curing anorectal cancer and restoring a good level of continence. Good quality of life may therefore be expected even in those patients whose cancer does not allow a sphincter-saving procedure. A short-term follow-up study shows that TAR supported by chronic electromyostimulation via implantable pulse generators may give an even better functional outcome.

Data from this study support the belief that with electrostimulated graciloplasty should be considered a safe and effective method to cure anorectal cancer without a need for a permanent abdominal stoma.

References

Abercrombie JE, Williams NS (1995) Total anorectal reconstruction. Br J Surg 82:438-442
Abulafi AM, Williams NS (1994) Local recurrence of colorectal cancer: the problem, mechanisms, management, and adjuvant therapy. Br J Surg 81:7-19
Baeten C, Spaans F, Fluks A (1988) An implanted neuromuscular stimulator for fecal continence following previously implanted gracilis muscle: report of a case. Dis Colon Rectum 31:134-137
Baeten CG, Konsten J, Spaans F et al (1991) Dynamic graciloplasty for treatment of fecal incontinence. Lancet 338:1163-1165
Beart RW, Steele GD, Menck HR et al (1995) Management and survival of patients with adenocarcinoma of the colon and rectum: a national survey of the Commission on Cancer. J Am Coll Surg 181:225-236
Berger A, Tiret E, Parc R et al (1992) Excision of the rectum with colonic J pouch - anal anastomosis for adenocarcinoma of the low and mid rectum. World J Surg 16:470-477.
Buess G, Mentges B, Manncke K et al (1992) Technique and results of transanal endoscopic microsurgery in early rectal cancer. Am J Surg 163:63-76
Cavina E (1996) Outcome of restorative perineal graciloplasty with simultaneous excision of the anus and the rectum for cancer. A ten-year experience with 81 patients. Dis Colon Rectum 39:182-190
Cavina E, Seccia M, Evangelista G (1981) Neossfintere e neostoma: nuove tecniche chirurgiche in funzione delle prospettive di elettrostimolazione per la continenza. Esperienza clinica. Min Chir 33:16-18
Cavina E, Seccia M, Evangelista G (1982) Neosphincter and neostomy. New surgical views for myoelectric stimulated continence. Preliminary report. Am J Proctol Gastroenterol Colon Rectum Surg 33:16-18
Cavina E, Seccia M, Evangelista et al (1987) Construction of a continent perineal colostomy by using electrostimulated gracilis muscles after abdominoperineal resection: personal technique and experience with 32 cases. Ital J Surg Sci 17:305-316
Cavina E, Seccia M, Evangelista G et al (1990) Perineal colostomy and electrostimulated gracilis neosphincter after abdominoperineal resection of the colon and anorectum. A surgical experience and follow-up study in 47 cases. Int J Colorectal Dis 5:6-11
Cavina E, Menconi C, Balestri R, Seccia M (1993) Static-dynamic graciloplasty: a reconstructive technique of the anal sphincter after abdominoperineal resection of the rectum. Dis Colon Rectum 36:29

Enker WE, Thaler HT, Cranor ML et al (1995) Total mesorectal excision in the treatment of carcinoma of the rectum. J Am Coll Surg 181:335-346

Geerdees BP, Zoetmulder FAN, Baeten CG (1995) Double dynamic graciloplasty and coloperineal pull-through after abdominoperineal resection. Eur J Cancer 31:1248-1252

Graf W, Påhlman L, Enblod P et al (1990) Anterior versus abdominoperineal resections in the management of mid-rectal tumours. Acta Chir Scand 156:231-235

Leo E, Belli F, Auderola S (1995) Total rectal resection, mesorectal excision and coloendoanal anastomosis: a therapeutic option for the treatment of low rectal cancer. Abstract Book, Int Conf on Rectal Cancer, Berlin, 29-30 September 1995

Mercati U, Trancanelli V, Castagnoli GP et al (1991) Use of the gracilis muscles for sphincteric construction after abdominoperineal resection. Technique and preliminary results. Dis Colon Rectum 34:1085-1089

Miles E (1908) A method of performing abdomino-perineal excision for carcinoma of the rectum and of the terminal portion of the pelvic colon. Lancet 2:1812-1813

Paty PB, Enker WE, Coehn AM et al (1994) Long-term functional results of coloanal anastomosis for rectal cancer. Am J Surg 167:91-95

Roseau E (1995) Reconstruction anorectal complète après amputation abdomino-périnéale du rectum. Presse Med24 (26):1189

Santoro E, Tirelli C, Scutari F et al (1994) Continent perineal colostomy by transposition of gracilis muscles. Dis Colon Rectum 37:173-179

Seccia M, Menconi C, Balestri R, Cavina E (1994) Study protocols and functional results in 86 electrostimulated graciloplasties. Dis Colon Rectum 37:897-904

Staimmer D, Kugler J (1995) Functional long-term results in the treatment of rectal carcinoma after coloanal anastomosis. Abstract Book, Int Conf on Rectal Cancer, Berlin, 29-30 September 1995

Sun WM, Read NW, Katsinelos P et al (1994) Anorectal function after restorative proctocolectomy and low anterior resection with coloanal anastomosis. Br J Surg 81:280-284

Williams NS (1992) Anorectal reconstruction. Br J Surg 79:733-734

Williams NS, Hallan RJ, Koeze TH, Watkins ES (1990) Restoration of gastrointestinal continuity and continence after abdominoperineal excision of the rectum using an electrically stimulated neoanal sphincter. Dis Colon Rectum 33:561-565

Local Excision of Rectal Cancer Through Windowed Specula: Long-Term Results

W. Slisow K. T. Moesta, P. M. Schlag

Department of Surgery and Surgical Oncology, Robert Rössle Hospital, Charité Humboldt University of Berlin, Lindenberger Weg 80, 13122 Berlin, Germany

Abstract

Transanal local excision of rectal cancer has been advocated as a curative option in patients with early rectal cancer and for patients unsuitable for radical surgery. We report our long-term experience with an easy-to-use and inexpensive technique based on windowed specula. From 1982 to 1994, 137 patients with rectal cancer were treated by local excision with curative intention. An R0 resection was possible in 74% of all patients and in 80% of the patients with a tumor surface of less than 9 cm^2. Ninety patients with a follow-up of more than 3 years (T1: $n=50$, T2: $n=30$, T3: $n=14$) were evaluated for survival. Seventy-four of these 90 patients are currently alive. The cause of death is known for all 16 deceased patients. In 4, death was tumor-related; 3 of these patients had a component of local failure. In 6 of 8 patients with local recurrence, a radical reresection was possible. The rate of recurrence increased with T category and with tumor grade. There has been one recurrence in a patient with a T1G1 cancer. The instrumentation enables adequate local excision of rectal cancers of less than 9 cm^2 surface area. In this group of patients including a considerable number with T2 and T3 cancers, only 3 died of tumor-related causes with a component of local failure, which compares well with mortality rates above 4% for abdominoperineal excision. Comparison with international data on radical surgery shows that the overall survival is not reduced by local transanal excision for early rectal cancer.

Introduction

Local excision of rectal cancer in the lower third of the rectum has long been advocated in very early lesions and in patients unsuitable for radical surgery [1–3]. The development of a transanal microsurgical technique by Buess et al. [4], facilitating full-thickness resection with adequate safety margins, has extended the indication to all low-grade, early cancers in the lower third of the rectum, regardless of the physical status of the patient, with the sole aim of sphincter preservation [5–7]. However, the popularity of the technique is limited by instrumentation that is expensive and difficult to handle [8]. Furthermore, there is still controversy about the indicational limits of the procedure.

At Robert Rössle Hospital, a former cancer care center of the former GDR, a proprietary, inexpensive, and easy-to-use technique was developed in 1982 enabling adequate local excision in the lower third of the rectum [9]. Unfortunately, this procedure has not obtained international attention due to inappropriate publication. We are now able to report long-term results.

Patients and Methods

Instrumentation and Procedure

A set of glass specula with closed tip and side windows of variable opening and position enables exposure of all rectal neoplasms situated in the lower and middle portions of the rectum (Fig. 1). The outer diameter of the specula varies from 4 to 5cm. The procedure is carried out in lithotomy position. The anal sphincter is carefully dilated by the cone-shaped tip of the specula. Once the appropriate speculum is in place, the lesion and a margin of surrounding mucosa protrude through the side window into the lumen, where full-thickness resection is performed with conventional instruments (Fig. 2).

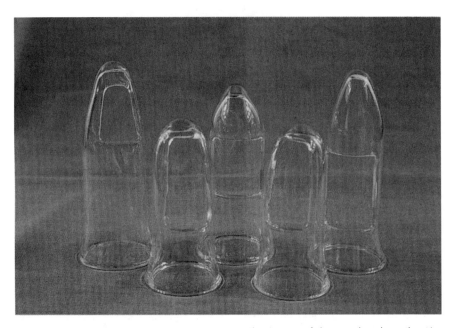

Fig. 1. Glass specula (Dewey) for transanal local excision. The diameter of the cone-shaped specula varies from 4–5 cm. Working windows of different size and position allow exposure of any tumor situated in the middle or lower rectum

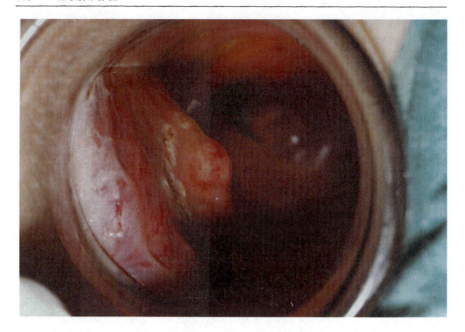

Fig. 2. The speculum in place, the tumor protrudes into the lumen of the device, where full-layer resection can be performed with conventional instrumentation

Lesions that exceed the window size are resected by sequentially exposing all parts of the tumor by rotation of the speculum. The closed tip of the speculum obliterates the bowel lumen and prevents spoilage of the surgical site. The resected specimen is pinned on cardboard under proper orientation by the surgeon himself (Fig. 3) for pathological evaluation.

Pathological Evaluation

A standard procedure is followed. The surgical specimen mounted on cardboard is measured, and the tumor surface is determined from two perpendicular diameters as (surface = diameter 1 × diameter 2) Serial sections are prepared at a distance of 2–3 mm and stained by hematoxylin and eosin. Infiltration depth, histological grade, and surgical radicality are classified according to the UICC TNM system, thus based on microscopic examination of the whole specimen in step sections each 2–3 mm apart.

Patients

Between 1982 and 1994, 137 patients (70 men and 67 women) with rectal cancer were treated by local excision with curative intention. Their mean age was 66.5 years (range 39–91). In 53/137 (39%) patients severe concomitant

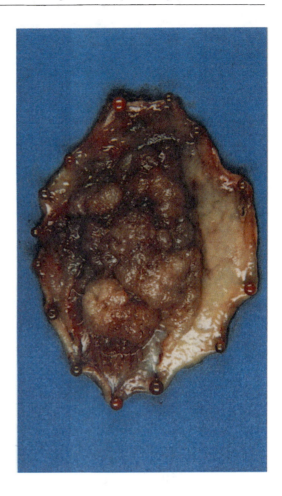

Fig. 3. Full-thickness resection specimen with a minimum of 5 mm margin, prepared and oriented by the surgeon for pathological analysis

disease was documented (ASA 3 or above). The procedure was indicated in early stage cancers for sphincter preservation or in patients with more advanced lesions and poor general health condition. Preoperative staging was determined by digital examination, and since 1989 by endorectal sonography. Patients with positive or indeterminable specimen margins were immediately reresected by a radical approach, or if the general health condition was poor, submitted to external radiation therapy. Standard follow-up was at 3-month intervals during the first 3 years, and twice yearly until 5 years.

Results

The histomorphological characteristics of the 137 rectal cancer specimens of patients resected under curative intention are presented in Table 1 and the age distribution of the patients in Fig. 4. Full-thickness resection was per-

Table 1. Morphological and histological characteristics of rectal cancers resected by transanal local excision for the total of 137 patients and for a subset of 90 patients with R0 resections

	All patients ($n=137$)		R0 resections ($n=90$)	
	n	%	n	%
Size (surface area)				
>3 cm^2	11	9	11	13
3–6 cm^2	29	24	22	26
6–9 cm^2	19	16	14	16
>9 cm^2	62	51	38	45
Infiltration depth				
pT1	64	47	50	56
pT2	49	36	27	30
pT3	23	17	13	14
Grading				
G1	73	53	50	56
G2	55	40	33	37
G3	10	7	7	8

Size is determined as the product of two perpendicular diameters on the freshly excised specimen (length and width, not depth). Size is available in 121/137 patients and in 85/90 R0-resected patients only, due to the retrospective nature of the study.

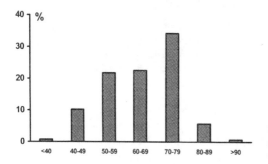

Fig. 4. Age distribution of 137 patients submitted to transanal resection of rectal cancer

formed in 79% of all cases; 13% of the resections were partial thickness, and 8% were mucosectomies. The resection was classified R0 in 74% of the patients and R1 in 12%. In 14% of the patients no reliable R classification was obtained, due mainly to mechanical alteration of the specimen during resection. The rate of R0 resections was considerably higher in tumors smaller than 9 cm^2 (80%, Fig. 5a) than in those larger than 9 cm^2 (62%, Fig. 5b).

Of the 101 patients with R0 resections 4 were lost to follow-up without evidence of recurrence between 1 year and 18 months after surgery. One patient died on the fourth postoperative day from massive pulmonary embolism. Four

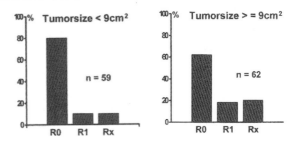

Fig. 5. Percentages of R0 resections in small and large tumors. *R0* Microscopically free resection margins; *R1*, resection margins microscopically involved by tumor; *Rx*, involvement of the specimens margins is uncertain, generally due to mechanical alteration of the specimen during resection. Radicality results for tumor surfaces (surface = product of two perpendicular diameters) smaller or larger than 9 cm^2

Table 2. Recurrences after transanal R0 resection of rectal cancer in 90 patients, according to T category, histological grading and specific combinations of both

	Recurrences	%
T category		
pT1	3/50	6
pT2	3/27	11
pT3a	2/13	16
Tumor grade		
G1	3/50	6
G2	3/33	9
G3	2/7	29
Constellations		
pT1 G1	1/30	3
pT1 G2	1/16	6
pT2 G1	1/15	7

patients were immediately reresected due to an underestimated tumor stage (patients suitable for radical surgery). A further two patients did not meet the criterion of at least 3 years follow-up in October 1997. The remaining 90 R0 resected patients with a follow-up of more than 3 years were evaluated for survival. Morphological and histological characteristics are presented in Table 1. The median follow-up is 5 years, and 85% of the patients have a follow-up of 5 years.

Overall survival is given in Fig. 6a. Of the 90 patients 74 are still alive. The cause of death is known for all of the 16 patients who died. Death was tumor-related in four (4.4% of the R0 resected patients over all stages). The tumor recurred locally in eight (9%) cases; in six of these the recurrence was only local while two also had a distant component. In six of the eight patients the local recurrence was again radically resectable (R0). One patient with unresectable local recurrence 42 months after the initial operation was

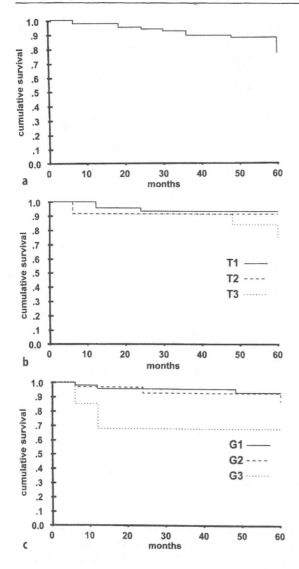

Fig. 6a–c. Survival in 90 patients after R0 local excision of rectal cancer. **a** Overall cumulative survival. **b** Disease-free survival according to T category *(T1–T3)*. **c** Disease free survival according to histological grade *(G1–G3)*

treated by external radiation and survived a total of 53 months. The second case, presenting with local recurrence and distant metastases at 51 months, received only supportive care and succumbed 58 months after initial surgery. One patient of the six reoperated upon for local recurrence was diagnosed with distant metastases 7 months after reoperation and died after a total survival of 15 months. Two others died of unrelated disease and the remaining three reoperated upon for local recurrence are disease-free (after 105, 85, and 63 months). One patient died after 73 months from liver metastases without evidence of local recurrence. Thus a total of 3/90 patients died of tumor-related causes with a component of local failure. The rate of recurrence increased with the T category and with tumor grade. There has been one recurrence among 30 pT1 G1 cancer patients and one in 16 pT1 G2 cancer patients (Table 2). Disease-free survival decreases with increasing T category (Fig. 6b) and with increasing tumor grade (Fig. 6b).

Discussion

Three factors have promoted local excisions in rectal cancer therapy: (a) the development of appropriate surgical techniques, (b) the increasing demand due to more effective early diagnosis, and (c) the availability of a reliable preoperative staging by endosonography. The development of appropriate transanal surgical technique made obsolete the posterior approach as a local procedure with higher morbidity and associated with considerable postoperative pain on sitting [10]. The highly sophisticated transanal endoscopic microsurgery developed by Buess et al. in 1983 [4] provides certainly the most precise technological approach. For economic reasons a number of conventional retractors are still used for the transanal approach, providing, however, inferior view and accessibility. The approach using urological resectoscopes as has been communicated by centers in the United Kingdom [11, 12] prevents proper pathological staging and is thus unacceptable. The windowed glass specula, while economically similar to typical retractor systems, provide good exposure with less sphincter distension than conventional retractors.

Transanal local excision is now a well-established treatment option for patients with low-grade T1 rectal cancer. Less-differentiated histologies, signs of vascular or lymph vessel invasion, and deeper infiltration of the bowel wall are considered contraindications for local excision. This is due mainly to the observation of an increased rate of lymphatic metastases associated with those factors [13-15]. In the analysis by Brodsky et al. [15] of 154 specimens of radical surgical resection in patients with T1 and T2 rectal cancers the rate of lymph node metastases rose from 12% in T1 tumors to 22% in T2 tumors, and from 0% (0/12) in grade 1 over 22% (23/106) in grade 2 to 50% (5/10) in grade 3 tumors (T1 and T2). Most remarkably, even in the subset of T1 grade 2 tumors, generally believed to be acceptable candidates for local excision, the rate of lymphatic micrometastases was 13% (2/15). With the occurrence of lymphatic or blood vessel invasion the incidence of lymphatic metastases rose from 17% to 31%. In good accordance with those numbers, Mentges et al. describe an increase in lymph node metastases with T category at reoperations after local excision [16]. Nine out of 64 T1 tumor patients were submitted to radical resections and none of them had evidence of lymphatic spread. Twenty of 33 local excisions revealing a T2 cancer were followed by radical procedure and revealed lymph node metastases in five cases. In ten reresections for T3 tumors two had lymphatic metastases.

The early institution of transanal resections and the historical situation of our hospital as the main referral center for the former GDR has led to a considerable number of patients being submitted only to local excision due to poor general condition. The more advanced tumor stages, in retrospect, do now allow the study of the natural course of such patients. The rate of 80% of R0 resections in tumors smaller than 9 cm^2 compares well with the results of the German Colorectal Carcinoma Study Group [17] for radical surgery of all stages. In view of the data presented above, it is most surprising that only 3 of 90 patients died from failure of local tumor control, 44 of whom would not meet the current criteria for local excision (pT1 G1:30/90; pT1 G2: 16/90). Of course, the rate of local recurrence increases with T category and with tumor grade. However, the majority (six of eight) of the local recurrences detected under appropriate follow-up were again suitable to radical surgery and were cured at a rate of 50%.

One explanation for these results may be that in a number of cases the directly adjacent lymph nodes are removed by our specific full-thickness approach. However, 36 patients of the original 137 were excluded from the analysis for involved or indeterminable margins. The rate of not-R0 resected cases increases with size. Thus, while size has never been shown to be an independent predictor of lymph node status, it may well be indirectly linked to established prognostic factors. If patients were therefore excluded from the study for a factor associated with a risk factor for lymphatic metastases, it is evident that the rate of lymphatic metastases in our study population may well be lower than that observed in unselected patient populations. In the series by Mentges et al. [16] 12 patients in the pT2 group were not submitted to radical reresection. While the rate of lymphatic metastases in the reresected T2 tumor patients was 25%, none of the patients who did not receive reresection developed a local recurrence (median follow-up of 29 months). Mentges et al. do not clearly state why certain patients in that group were reresected and others were not; again, some selection may have also taken place at this point.

In view of a mortality of the abdominoperineal excision, which exceeds the 3.3% of local treatment associated failures (German Colorectal Carcinoma Study Group [17]: 4.3% total operative mortality), it seems warranted to extend the indication of local excision to low-grade T2 and in selected cases with impaired general condition even to early T3 low-grade tumors. However, at least with our type of procedure we emphasize an upper size limit of 9 cm^2. Patients with involved or indeterminable margins must undergo radical reresection or radiation therapy.

References

1. Lock MR (1990) Fifty years of local excision for rectal carcinoma. Ann R Coll Surg Engl 72:170–171
2. Killingback MJ (1985) Indications for local excision of rectal cancer. Br J Surg 72 Suppl:S54–56
3. Hager T, Gall FP, Hermanek P (1983) Local excision of cancer of the rectum. Dis Colon Rectum 26:149–151

4. Buess G, Theiss R, Hutterer F, Pichlmaier H, Pelz C, Holfeld T, Said S, Isselhard W (1983) Die transanale endoskopische Rektumoperation - Erprobung einer neuen Methode im Tierversuch. Leber Magen Darm 13:73-77
5. Banerjee AK, Jehle EC, Shorthouse AJ, Buess G (1995) Local excision of rectal tumours. Br J Surg 82:1165-1173
6. Steele RJ, Hershman MJ, Mortensen NJ, Armitage NC, Scholefield JH (1996) Transanal endoscopic microsurgery-initial experience from three centres in the United Kingdom. Br J Surg 83:207-210
7. Lezoche E, Guerrieri M, Paganini A Feliciotti F, Di Pietrantonj F (1996) Is transanal endoscopic microsurgery (TEM) a valid treatment for rectal tumors? Surg Endosc 10:736-741
8. Swanstrom LL, Smiley P, Zelko J, Cagle L (1997) Video endoscopic transanal-rectal tumor excision. Am J Surg 173:383-385
9. Dewey P, Seifart W (1985) Geschlossenes und seitlich gefenstertes Spekulum zur peranalen Tumorexstirpation. Zentralbl Chir 110:43-45
10. Huber PJ Jr, Reiss G (1993) Rectal tumors: treatment with a posterior approach. Am J Surg 166:760-763
11. Courtney SP, Nankivell C, Davidson CM (1991) Endoscopic transanal resection of rectal lesions: facilitation by adaptation of Lord's dilator. J R Coll Surg Edinb 36:249-250
12. Dickinson AJ, Savage AP, Mortensen NJ, Kettlewell MG (1993) Long-term survival after endoscopic transanal resection of rectal tumours. Br J Surg 80:1401-1404
13. Saclarides TJ, Bhattacharyya AK, Britton Kuzel C, Szeluga D, Economou SG (1994) Predicting lymph node metastases in rectal cancer. Dis Colon Rectum 37:52-57
14. Slisow W, Kolbow C, Fischer J (1993) Perioperative klinisch-pathomorphologische Beurteilung des pararektalen Lymphknotenstatus und ihr Beitrag zur definitiven Entscheidung für eine lokale Exstirpation des Rektumkarzinoms. Zentralbl Chir 118:197-202
15. Brodsky JT, Richard GK, Cohen AM, Minsky BD (1992) Variables correlated with the risk of lymph node metastasis in early rectal cancer. Cancer 69:322-326
16. Mentges B, Buess G, Effinger G, Manncke K, Becker HD (1997) Indications and results of local treatment of rectal cancer. Br J Surg 84:348-351
17. Kessler H, Hermanek P Jr, Wiebelt H (1993) Operative mortality in carcinoma of the rectum. Results of the German Multicentre Study. Int J Colorectal Dis 8:158-166

Prevention of Local Recurrence

Locoregional Recurrence of Rectal Cancer: Biological and Technical Aspects of Surgical Failure

P. Hohenberger

Department of Surgery and Surgical Oncology, Robert Rössle Hospital, Charité Humboldt University of Berlin, Lindenberger Weg 80, 13125 Berlin, Germany

Abstract

The advantages of sphincter-saving treatment of rectal cancer are counterbalanced when local recurrences develop requiring abdominal-perineal excision of the rectum for salvage. Biological properties of the primary tumor contribute to this problem together with the surgeon's technique and overall oncological strategy. Adverse factors of the primary tumor are lymphatic, perineural, and venous invasion as well as mucinous type of adenocarcinoma and poor differentiation. Although tumor cells can adhere to suture material there is not sufficient evidence that the suture material contributes significantly to local relapse. Intraoperative tumor cell spillage is often provoked by the surgeon's technique in handling the tumor and the non-use of methods to prevent the seeding of exfoliated cells. Adequate operative techniques such as complete mesorectal excision, washing of rectal stump, and complete eradication of lymphatic spread of the tumor are prerequisites for low recurrence rates. Distal margins of clearance alone are of less importance than expected previously. Surgeons are the leaders in taking care of patients suffering from rectal cancer and they must apply their knowledge of tumor biological factors to their operative technique to avoid local recurrence of tumors.

Introduction

A variety of surgical techniques make it possible to maintain the anal sphincter by performing a low or ultra-low anastomosis or to restore continence via different types of muscular reconstructions. However, the advantages of sphincter-saving treatment of rectal cancer are counterbalanced when a local recurrence develops and abdominoperineal excision is required as a salvage procedure.

Unfortunately, the incidence of local recurrence following rectal cancer treatment remains high (Table 1). Recent series reporting data from well-conducted clinical trials such as the Large Bowel Cancer Project (LBCP) in the United Kingdom and the North Central Cancer Treatment Group (NCCTG)

Table 1. Incidence of local recurrences after treatment for colorectal cancer reported in multicenter studies from experienced cooperative groups

Study	n	Recurrence rate
Phillips et al. (1984a) LBCP, Great Britain	1052	14%
Krook et al. (1991) NCCTG trial	204	13% vs. 25%
Galandiuk et al. (1992) adjuvant trials	818	21%
Sause et al. (1994) RTOG 81–15	353	26%

and the Radiation Therapy Oncology Group (RTOG) in the United States document recurrence rates between 13% and 26% (Sause et al. 1994; Galandiuk et al. 1992; Krook et al. 1991; Phillips et al. 1984a).

Factors affecting locoregional recurrence rates include the tumor and its biological properties and the surgeon. The surgical contribution to failure may be related to the surgeon's operative technique, overall oncological strategy, and the device used for anastomosis.

Biological Properties of the Tumor Contributing to Locoregional Recurrence

Several characteristics of the primary tumor are correlated with an increased local regional recurrence rate. Lymph node metastases, lymphangiosis carcinomatosa, and arterial or venous invasion are well-documented influencing factors (Horn et al. 1991; Bognel et al. 1995) represented by the TNM system (N+, L1, V1). Also, poor differentiation of the tumor (grade 3/4) has regularly been shown to be overrepresented in patients with local failure, as seen in our own series of local treatment (Slisow/Schlag, this volume) or the series reported by Marks (this volume).

Further aspects of the tumor biology of primary rectal cancer have to be considered. In particular subtypes of rectal cancer the risk of lymph node metastases may be high. Heald and coworkers examined 109 resection specimens of low rectal cancer and assessed a minimum of 13 lymph nodes histopathologically. Even in rectal cancers confined to the submucosa (pT1 tumors), in up to 11% of cases lymph nodes occupied by tumor were found. In tumors with poor differentiation (grade 3), lymph node metastases were detected in up to 42% of the resection specimens (Huddy et al. 1993).

Mucinous adenocarcinomas are reported to be overrepresented in pT3/4 tumors, in contrast to tumors with less local infiltration (pT1/2 tumors). Additionally, this tumor type shows a higher incidence of lymph node metastases as well as a greater ratio of regional recurrences than nonmucinous adenocarcinomas (Hohenberger et al. 1992; Okuno et al. 1988; Umpleby et al.

1985). A decreased survival rate after the treatment of a recurrence was also observed.

Interaction Between Tumor Cells and Suture Material

It was assumed that suture material could contribute to the incidence of locoregional recurrences (Reinbach et al. 1993; Phillips and Cook 1986; Hurst et al. 1982). A tumor relapse at the anastomosis represents a distinct entity, and different subtypes have been described (Umpleby and Williamson 1987). The tumor extension may be confined to the mucosa, may involve both mucosa and rectal wall, or may develop predominantly from an extraluminal site with invasion to the lumen. Suture material sometimes can be detected within the recurrence (Fig. 1), and the question arises whether this is causative.

Reports from animal models and tumor cell cultures suggest a different adherence of tumor cells to silk, steel, or polyglycol sutures (Table 2). Less favorable results were obtained when steel wires were used, but no influence of the technique of their insertion could be demonstrated (Phillips and Cook 1986). These findings were questioned by McGregor et al. (1991), who could not demonstrate a significant difference in tumor formation at the anastomosis with different suturing materials in the postinitiating phase of carcinogenesis in a rat model. However, later the same group reported a highly significant difference of adhesion of intraperitoneal tumor cells to longitudinal

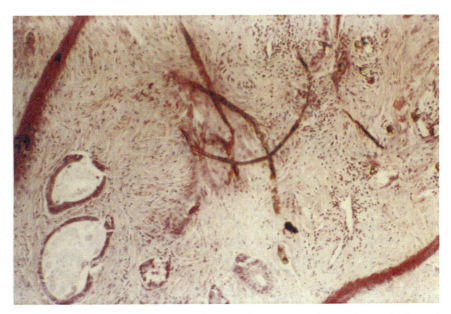

Fig. 1. Suture material within a local recurrence located at the anastomosis after anterior resection for rectal cancer

Table 2. Affinity and adhesion of tumor cells in a rat animal model to sutur material used for anastomoses in rectal cancer surgery. Data from Phillips et al. (1986), McGregor et al. (1991), Reinbach et al. (1993)

	Adherence	Implantation
Prolene		–
Steel wire	–	–
Chromic catgut		+
Polyamide	+	
Nylon		+
Silk		++
Polyglycol	++	+++

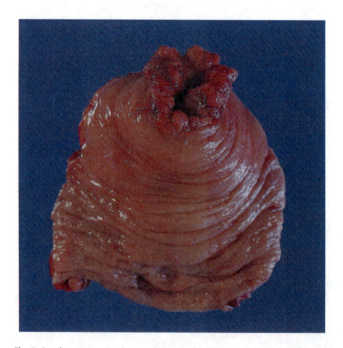

Fig. 2. Local recurrence in the rectal stump after Hartmann's procedure for rectal cancer

colotomies depending on the type of suture material used (Reinbach et al. 1993). Summarizing the data, it cannot be concluded that anastomoses resulting from stapling machines using stainless steel clamps really bear a higher risk of local recurrence, as was initially suspected (Hurst et al. 1982).

The *surgical wound* itself must be considered as a factor when discussing factors contributing to local failure. In a mouse model with circulating tumor cells after resection of the primary tumor, the overwhelming majority of recurrences were at the skin incision. Radiotherapy to the incision line was unable to prevent the formation of tumor deposits. The results of a cell dilution assay suggested 39 tumor cells to be enough to initiate the relapse (Baker et al. 1989). This mechanism may account for the typical sites of implantation metastases at the abdominal wall (Ledesma et al. 1982), the perineum, the colostomy, or the rectal stump in the case of Hartman's procedure (Fig. 2). Inoculation with viable tumor cells takes place during the operation and will not be recognized by the surgeon in the overwhelming majority of cases. Taking into consideration recent results from peritoneal cytology and bone marrow biopsies (Juhl et al. 1994; O'Sullivan et al. 1995) as methods for assessing tumor spread, it must be assumed that tumor cells are spilled into the operation field on resection of tumors with invasion beyond the rectal wall or occupation of regional lymph nodes.

Locoregional Tumor Spread and the Surgeon's Operative Approach

Another means of tumor propagation has to be taken into account - endo- or perineural invasion (Fig. 3). Multivariate analysis revealed that even pT2 tumors are associated with neural invasion in about 10% and pT3/4 tumors in up to 50% of cases (Bognel et al. 1995). Obviously, this phenomenon derives from a specific capability of tumor cells to invade neural sheaths (Kenmotsu et al. 1994; Wimmenauer et al. 1997; Seki et al. 1995). A significant influence on disease-free survival has been reported (Krasna et al. 1988; Horn

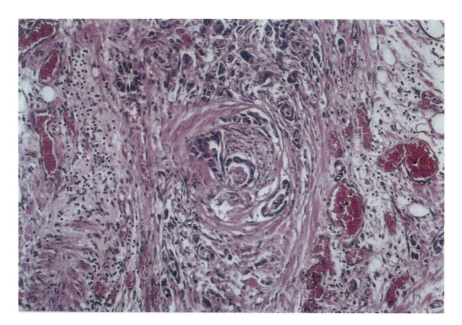

Fig. 3. Invasion of the perineural sheaths by adenocarcinoma of the rectum

et al. 1991; Bognel et al. 1995). However, this may be affected not only by tumor biological properties but also by the surgical technique.

The *genitourinary morbidity* after anterior resection is rather high (Harnsberger et al. 1994; Hojo et al. 1991). Sexual impotence is reported by up to 56% of the patients. Urinary dysfunction is present in the form of incontinence in 44% and pollakisuria in 59% of the patients followed up after conventional anterior resection. In contrast, *nerve-sparing surgery* can decrease sexual dysfunction rates to 27%, urinary incontinence to 22%, and pollakisuria to 24% (Cosimelli et al. 1994; Koukouras et al. 1991). In a series of more than 300 patients the 5-year disease-free survival rate was 58.5%, but the local recurrence rate even in the favourable stages was at least 11.5%.

Maintaining sexual function and avoiding urinary dysfunction during mesorectal clearance is a very important goal (Havenga et al. 1996). Tumor spread within perineural sheaths and its influence on local recurrence, however, requires a thorough discussion whether the price of a patient being happy with maintenance of sexual function is not an increased risk of local recurrence.

Tumor Cell Spillage and Implantation Metastases

As pointed out earlier, even a minimum of viable tumor cells spilled into the operation field may result in recurrent tumor growth (Hansen et al. 1995). Tumor cell spillage can occur intraperitoneally, inside the lymphatics, within the lumen of the colon and rectum, or intravasally. This may result in micrometastases to the liver and lung, circulating tumor cells to the blood, or cytokeratin-positive cells in the bone marrow (O'Sullivan et al. 1995). The presence of viable tumor cells at the site of intestinal anastomoses supports their potential role in the etiology of suture-line recurrences.

Recurrence at the anastomosis as an entity of locoregional relapse is less often observed nowadays (Umpleby et al. 1984, 1987; Hohenberger et al. 1992). The chance for a R0 resection of this type of recurrence is higher than in other forms of tumor relapse and the median survival thereafter is in general more favorable. In the early 1980s, the first experience with the use of staplers to create low rectal anastomoses was followed by reports of increased local recurrence rates (Hurst et al. 1982). Umpleby and co-workers demonstrated that within the colon lumen viable cells are exfoliated during manipulation for primary tumor resection in 70% of the specimens (Umpleby et al. 1984). The number of viable tumor cells did not correlate with the stage or differentiation of the tumor. However, the number of tumor cells recovered from the distal resection margin was inversely related to the distance of the tumor from that margin.

These cells can adhere to the anastomosis and re-grow as a tumor recurrence. McCue and Phillips (1993) postulated an increased cell turnover at the anastomosis and a promotional effect on tumor growth. However, as could be shown from the interference of suture material with tumor recurrence, steel suture clamps of staplers do not favor local recurrences. It is therefore not the device that is responsible for an increased recurrence rate, but surgeons performing more "risky" operations because they feel that the new device expands their technical facilities or they do not use methods to prevent intraoperative tumor cell spillage.

Inadvertent perforation or incision of a rectal carcinoma during surgery may lead to massive dissemination of tumor cells in the operative area. This was observed in up to 8.7% of 1360 radical resections for cure. Local recurrence was seen in 39% of cases of spillage of tumor cells. Intraoperative tumor cell spillage has a negative effect on survival rates, reducing the 5-year survival rate after resection with curative intent from 70% to 44% (Zirngibl et al. 1990).

Surgical Oncology Strategy

Although the biological properties of the primary tumor greatlly influence the risk of recurrence, adequate adjuvant treatment postoperatively must form part of the overall oncological strategy. It has been proven that radiochemotherapy after resection of rectal cancer beyond the rectal wall or with lymph node metastases may reduce the incidence of local failure (Krook et al. 1991). Thus, particularly patients whose tumor expresses unfavorable histological criteria should be scheduled for adjuvant treatment. The selected postoperative therapy should be capable of counteracting the increased risk of local relapse. An increased local recurrence rate in patients not subjected to additional treatment is due to failure in the surgical oncologist's strategy, omitting adjuvant treatment of proven efficacy.

Discusison with the patient whether combined modality therapy is advisable is particularly important if limited resection is being considered for early rectal cancer [e.g. local excision with or without radiotherapy (Willett et al. 1994)] or in the case of la ocally advanced tumor. Neoadjuvant treatment concepts for T3 or T4 rectal cancer showed better results than postoperative strategies with respect to morbidity, downstaging, and local recurrence rates (Pahlman, this volume; Riess et al. 1995; Minsky et al. 1992).

Factors Influencing Local Tumor Relapse: Historical Aspects

The discussion of ways to avoid local tumor relapse after surgery for rectal cancer has continued throughout this century, with topics changing and various approaches being advanced. Controversy whether anterior resection could result in identical recurrence rates was common until the 1970s. The next major topics were the distal margin of clearance (Hermanek and Gall 1981; Goligher 1951) and the influence of the so-called no-touch isolation technique (Turnbull 1975). Later on, histological typing and grading attracted major interest, followed by the influence of using the stapling gun for anastomoses. Within the past 10-15 years the complete eradication of the mesorectum and lateral clearance have been debated (Heald et al. 1982). Most recently, clear evidence has emerged that the individual surgeon has considerable influence on recurrence rates and survival in rectal cancer surgery (Hermanek et al. 1994; McArdle et al. 1990; Phillips et al. 1984b).

Aspects of Operative Technique Contributing to Local Tumor Relapse

The surgical aspects of locoregional failure relate to the different steps during anterior resection or abdominoperineal excision:
- High versus low ligation of the arterial blood supply
- Distal length of clearance
- Lateral spread of tumor
- Complete mesorectal excision
- Washing of the rectal stump
- Nerve-sparing resection technique (mentioned above).

Dissection of the Lymphatic Drainage Area

The question of high or low ligation of the inferior mesenteric artery has ben addressed several times. Moynihan (1908) and Turnbull et al. (1967) were strong advocates of the more radical approach, recommending ligation of the inferior mesenteric artery close to the aorta. However, four randomized trials (Corder et al. 1992; Surtees et al. 1990; Wiggers et al. 1988; Pezim and Nicholls 1984) failed to show a significant advantage regarding patients' survival, although decreased locoregional recurrence rates were observed.

In our experience, 30 patients presented with a regional recurrence after left hemicolectomy or anterior resection. Twenty-one of them showed residual nodes at the inferior mesenteric artery or the superior rectal artery being infiltrated by tumor (Hohenberger et al. 1991). This type of recurrence has characteristic features: the patient is asymptomatic with rising CEA and uneventful colonoscopy, and the diagnosis is made by endoluminal ultrasound or CT. Angiography of the inferior mesenteric artery detects the lymphatic recurrence by demonstrating the remaining blood supply. The low number of lymph nodes in the prior resection specimen of the primary tumor is another indicator of regional lymphatic recurrence due to incomplete dissection of mesosigmoid and mesorectal lymph nodes. As this type of recurrence might be re-resected with curative intent, the question arises whether adequate dissection of the lymphatics should not in fact take place during the operation for the primary tumor.

The history of complete lymphatic recurrence started in 1908, when Clogg stated that "any operation for cancer is not merely the removal of the primary growth but also of its lymphatics". Westhues in 1934 very carefully examined the lymphatic spread of colorectal cancer and formulated prerequi-

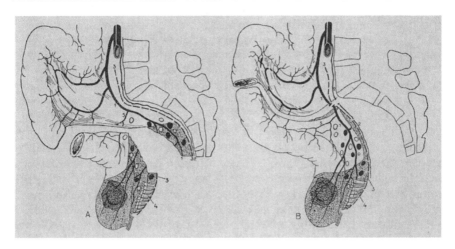

Fig. 4. Regional recurrence of rectal cancer due to inadequate clearance of the lymphatics. From Westhues (1934)

Table 3. Treatment results prior to and after adopting total mesorectal clearance in different hospitals data from (Enker et al. 1995; Volpe et al. 1996; Arbman et al. 1996; Aitken 1996)

	Before	After
Arbman et al. (1996) Norrköping	14	6.5
Enker et al. (1995) Sloan Kettering	28	7.3
Aitken (1996) Edinburgh	–	1
Volpe et al. (1996) Roswell Park	16	7.1

sites for an ideal operative specimen. He compared different techniques for rectal excision (the Kraske versus the Götze approach; Fig. 4) with respect to the lymph nodes left behind. Although his analysis of recurrent tumors did not detect the mesorectum as the entity to drain the lymphatics from the rectum, Westhues recommended accurate dissection of the lymphatics.

About 50 years later, Heald pointed out that the mesorectum was the "clue to pelvic recurrence" in rectal cancer surgery and accurately demonstrated that with adequate operative technique local recurrence rates of about 5% or less can be achieved (Heald et al. 1982, 1986). Heald's promotion of the distribution of his experience by teaching colleagues in the UK, Sweden, Germany, and the US must be seen as the major contribution to rectal cancer surgery in the last decade. Dramatic changes in local recurrence rate were reported by those adopting to his technique (Table 3) (Volpe et al. 1996; Aitken 1996; Enker et al. 1995; Arbman et al. 1996).

Distal Margins of Clearance

The history of distal margins of clearance over the past 50 years is also very interesting. The first approach was that all tumors growing beyond the coulter sac should be treated by abdominoperineal excision. Later, a distal resection margin of at least 5 cm seemed mandatory when performing an anterior resection (Goligher 1951; Grinnell 1965). Later on, a margin of at least 3 cm on the non-extended fresh resection specimen was regarded sufficient (Hermanek and Gall 1981; Tonak et al. 1982). In recent years, Quirke and coworkers have examined the role of lateral tumor spread and circumferential margin involvement with respect to local recurrence-free survival. After their initial paper in 1986, they were able to demonstrate that intra- and extramural recurrences often arise in patients with incompletely resected lateral tumor spread. The specific technique of slicing the resection specimen into coronal sections of the tumor and mesorectum not only allows examination of the axial tumor growth but evaluates completeness of lateral clearance (Adam et al. 1994; Scott et al. 1995). They could show that circumferential spread was a negative prognostic factor in both Dukes' B and C lesions. These findings indicated another site to be cleared by the surgeon; the distal resection margin seemed less important than complete eradication of tumor spread to the lateral pelvis, and so-called close-shave resections have been advocated (Karanjia et al. 1990).

In conjunction with complete mesorectal excision as advocated by Heald, both aspects of surgical technique contribute in convincing manner to the extremely low incidence of local recurrences now reported (Table 3).

Treatment of the Rectal Stump Before and During Anterior Resection

Besides complete dissection of the lymphatics, attention must be paid to avoiding spillage of tumor cells to the rectal stump when performing anterior resection. Some type of washing seems to be mandatory, irrespective of the technique used for anastomosis. As mentioned earlier, viable tumor cells can be detected in the lumen of the colorectum, leading to implantation metastases at the anastomosis. After so-called low anterior resection (median location of tumor 12.6 cm above anal verge), cells classified as Pap IV were found in 9 out of 10 washings of the rectal stump (Gertsch et al. 1992). Numerous cytotoxic agents are available to kill malignant cells exfoliated into the colorectal lumen (Umpleby and Williamson 1984).

Conclusion

Most of the factors contributing to locoregional recurrence of the rectal cancer have been analyzed over recent decades. Questions on abdominoperineal excision versus anterior resection and concerning the distal margin of clearance have been raised and answered. The no-touch isolation technique has been introduced and shown to decrease the incidence of recurrences but not to influence survival. Stapling devices facilitate total mesorectal excision and help to achieve clear lateral margins, in addition to maintaining anal continence.

The surgeon has to consider this knowledge of tumor biological factors in deciding on his or her personal operative technique. The daily practical routine must be adapted accordingly. To adhere to the rules of oncological surgery in terms of no-touch isolation, total mesorectal clearance is mandatory, but also surgical efforts must be combined with those of medical oncology or radiation therapy. The surgeon, as the leader in taking care of rectal cancer patients, remains the person primarily responsible for improving the still disappointing local recurrence rates.

References

Adam IJ, Mohamdee MO, Martin IG, Scott N, Finan PJ, Johnston D, Dixon MF, Quirke P (1994) Role of circumferential margin involvement in the local recurrence of rectal cancer. Lancet 344:707–711

Aitken RJ (1996) Mesorectal excision for rectal cancer. Br J Surg 83:214–216

Arbman G, Nilsson E, Hallbook O, Sjodahl R (1996) Local recurrence following total mesorectal excision for rectal cancer. Br J Surg 83:375–379

Baker DG, Masterson TM, Pace R, Constable WC, Wanebo H (1989) The influence of the surgical wound on local tumor recurrence. Surgery 106:525–532

Bognel C, Rekacewicz C, Mankarios H, Pignon JP, Elias D, Duvillard P, Prade M, Ducreux M, Kac J, Rougier P, et al (1995) Prognostic value of neural invasion in rectal carcinoma: a multivariate analysis on 339 patients with curative resection. Eur J Cancer 31A:894–898

Clogg HS (1908) Cancer of the colon. A study of 72 cases. Lancet II:1007–1011

Corder AP, Karanjia ND, Williams JD, Heald RJ (1992) Flush aortic tie versus selective preservation of the ascending left colic artery in low anterior resection for rectal carcinoma. Br J Surg 79:680–682

Cosimelli M, Mannella E, Giannarelli D, Casaldi V, Wappner G, Cavaliere F, Consolo S, Appetecchia M, Cavaliere R (1994) Nerve-sparing surgery in 302 resectable rectosigmoid cancer patients: genitourinary morbidity and 10-year survival. Dis Colon Rectum 37:S42–46

Enker WE, Thaler HT, Cranor ML, Polyak T (1995) Total mesorectal excision in the operative treatment of carcinoma of the rectum. J Am Coll Surg 181:335–346

Galandiuk S, Wieand HS, Moertel CG, Cha SS, Fitzgibbons RJ Jr., Pemberton JH, Wolff BG (1992) Patterns of recurrence after curative resection of carcinoma of the colon and rectum. Surg Gynecol Obstet 174:27–32

Gertsch P, Baer HU, Kraft R, Maddern GJ, Altermatt HJ (1992) Malignant cells are collected on circular staplers. Dis Colon Rectum 35:238–241

Goligher JC (1951) Local recurrences after sphincter-saving excisions for carcinoma of the rectum and rectosigmoid. Br J Surg 39:199–211

Grinnell R (1965) Results of ligation of inferior mesenteric artery at the aorta in resections of carcinoma of the descending colon and rectum. Surg Gynecol Obstet 114:1031

Hansen E, Wolff N, Knuechel R, Ruschoff J, Hofstaedter F, Taeger K (1995) Tumor cells in blood shed from the surgical field. Arch Surg 130:387–393

Harnsberger JR, Vernava VM, Longo WE (1994) Radical abdominopelvic lymphadenectomy: historic perspective and current role in the surgical management of rectal cancer. Dis Colon Rectum 37:73–87

Havenga K, Enker WE, McDermott K, Cohen AM, Minsky BD, Guillem J (1996) Male and female sexual and urinary function after total mesorectal excision with autonomic nerve preservation for carcinoma of the rectum. J Am Coll Surg 182:495-502

Heald RJ, Ryall RD (1986) Recurrence and survival after total mesorectal excision for rectal cancer. Lancet 1:1479-1482

Heald RJ, Husband EM, Ryall RD (1982) The mesorectum in rectal cancer surgery - the clue to pelvic recurrence? Br J Surg 69:613-616

Hermanek P, Gall FP (1981) Safe aboral distance in the sphincter-preserving resection of the rectum. Chirurg 52:25-29

Hermanek P Jr, Wiebelt H, Riedl S, Staimmer D, Hermanek P (1994) Long-term results of surgical therapy of colon cancer. Results of the Colorectal Cancer Study Group. Chirurg 65:287-297

Hohenberger P, Schlag P, Kretzschmar U, Herfarth C (1991) Regional mesenteric recurrence of colorectal cancer after anterior resection or left hemicolectomy: inadequate primary resection demonstrated by angiography of the remaining arterial supply. Int J Colorectal Dis 6:17-23

Hohenberger P, Schlag P, Herfarth C (1992) Reoperation in colorectal carcinoma with curative intention. Schweiz Med Wochenschr 122:1079-1086

Hojo K, Vernava AM 3d, Sugihara K, Katumata K (1991) Preservation of urine voiding and sexual function after rectal cancer surgery. Dis Colon Rectum 34:532-539

Horn A, Dahl O, Morild I (1991) Venous and neural invasion as predictors of recurrence in rectal adenocarcinoma. Dis Colon Rectum 34:798-804

Huddy SP, Husband EM, Cook MG, Gibbs NM, Marks CG, Heald RJ (1993) Lymph node metastases in early rectal cancer. Br J Surg 80:1457-1458

Hurst PA, Prout WG, Kelly JM, Bannister JJ, Walker RT (1982) Local recurrence after low anterior resection using the staple gun. Br J Surg 69:275-276

Juhl H, Stritzel M, Wroblewski A, Henne Bruns D, Kremer B, Schmiegel W, Neumaier M, Wagener C, Schreiber HW, Kalthoff H (1994) Immunocytological detection of micrometastatic cells: comparative evaluation of findings in the peritoneal cavity and the bone marrow of gastric, colorectal and pancreatic cancer patients. Int J Cancer 57:330-335

Karanjia ND, Schache DJ, North WR, Heald RJ (1990) 'Close shave' in anterior resection. Br J Surg 77:510-512

Kenmotsu M, Gouchi A, Maruo Y, Murashima N, Hiramoto Y, Iwagaki H, Orita K (1994) The expression of neural cell adhesion molecule (NCAM), neural invasion and recurrence patterns in rectal cancer - a study using anti-NACM (neural cell adhesion molecule) antibody. Nippon Geka Gakkai Zasshi 95:66-70

Koukouras D, Spiliotis J, Scopa CD, Dragotis K, Kalfarentzos F, Tzoracoleftherakis E, Androulakis J (1991) Radical consequence in the sexuality of male patients operated for colorectal carcinoma. Eur J Surg Oncol 17:285-288

Krasna MJ, Flancbaum L, Cody RP, Shneibaum S, Ben Ari G (1988) Vascular and neural invasion in colorectal carcinoma. Incidence and prognostic significance. Cancer 61:1018-1023

Krook JE, Moertel CG, Gunderson LL, Wieand HS, Collins RT, Beart RW, Kubista TP, Poon MA, Meyers WC, Mailliard JA (1991) Effective surgical adjuvant therapy for high-risk rectal carcinoma. N Engl J Med 324:709-715

Ledesma EJ, Tseng M, Mittelman A (1982) Surgical treatment of isolated abdominal wall metastasis in colorectal cancer. Cancer 50:1884-1887

McArdle CS, Hole D, Hansell D, Blumgart LH, Wood CB (1990) Prospective study of colorectal cancer in the west of Scotland: 10-year follow-up. Br J Surg 77:280-282

McCue JL, Phillips RK (1993) Cellular proliferation at sutured and sutureless colonic anastomoses. Dis Colon Rectum 36:468-474

McGregor JR, Galloway DJ, Jarrett F, Brown IL, George WD (1991) Anastomotic suture materials and experimental colorectal carcinogenesis. Dis Colon Rectum 34:987-992

Minsky BD, Cohen AM, Kemeny N, Enker WE, Kelsen DP, Reichman B, Saltz L, Sigurdson ER, Frankel J (1992) Enhancement of radiation-induced downstaging of rectal cancer by fluorouracil and high-dose leucovorin chemotherapy. J Clin Oncol 10:79-84

Moynihan BGA (1908) The surgical treatment of cancer of the sigmoid flexure and rectum with special reference to the principles to be observed. Surg Gynecol Obstet 6:463

O'Sullivan GC, Collins JK, O'Brien F, Crowley B, Murphy K, Lee G, Shanahan F (1995) Micrometastases in bone marrow of patients undergoing "curative" surgery for gastrointestinal cancer. Gastroenterology 109:1535-1540

Okuno M, Ikehara T, Nagayama M, Kato Y, Yui S, Umeyama K (1988) Mucinous colorectal carcinoma: clinical pathology and prognosis. Am Surg 54:681-685

Pezim ME, Nicholls RJ (1984) Survival after high or low ligation of the inferior mesenteric artery during curative surgery for rectal cancer. Ann Surg 200:729-733

Phillips RK, Cook HT (1986) Effect of steel wire sutures on the incidence of chemically induced rodent colonic tumours. Br J Surg 73:671-674

Phillips RK, Hittinger R, Blesovsky L, Fry JS, Fielding LP (1984a) Local recurrence following 'curative' surgery for large bowel cancer. II. The rectum and rectosigmoid. Br J Surg 71:17-20

Phillips RK, Hittinger R, Blesovsky L, Fry JS, Fielding LP (1984b) Large bowel cancer: surgical pathology and its relationship to survival. Br J Surg 71:604-610

Quirke P, Durdey P, Dixon MF, Williams NS (1986) Local recurrence of rectal adenocarcinoma due to inadequate surgical resection. Histopathological study of lateral tumour spread and surgical excision. Lancet 2:996-999

Reinbach D, McGregor JR, O'Dwyer PJ (1993) Effect of suture material on tumour cell adherence at sites of colonic injury. Br J Surg 80:774-776

Riess H, Loffel J, Wust P, Rau B, Gremmler M, Speidel A, Schlag P (1995) A pilot study of a new therapeutic approach in the treatment of locally advanced stages of rectal cancer: neoadjuvant radiation, chemotherapy and regional hyperthermia. Eur J Cancer 31A:1356-1360

Sause WT, Pajak TF, Noyes RD, Dobelbower R, Fischbach RJ, Doggett S, Mohiuddin M (1994) Evaluation of preoperative radiation therapy in operable colorectal cancer. Ann Surg 220:668-675

Scott N, Jackson P, al Jaberi T, Dixon MF, Quirke P, Finan PJ (1995) Total mesorectal excision and local recurrence: a study of tumour spread in the mesorectum distal to rectal cancer. Br J Surg 82:1031-1033

Seki H, Koyama K, Tanaka J, Sato Y, Umezawa A (1995) Neural cell adhesion molecule and perineural invasion in gallbladder cancer. J Surg Oncol 58:97-100

Surtees P, Ritchie JK, Phillips RK (1990) High versus low ligation of the inferior mesenteric artery in rectal cancer. Br J Surg 77:618-621

Tonak J, Gall FP, Hermanek P, Hager TH (1982) Incidence of local recurrence after curative operations for cancer of the rectum. Aust N Z J Surg 52:23-27

Turnbull RB Jr (1975) Current concepts in cancer. Cancer of the GI tract: colon, rectum, anus. The no-touch isolation technique of resection. JAMA 231:1181-1182

Turnbull RB Jr, Kyle K, Watson FR, Spratt J (1967) Cancer of the colon: the influence of the no-touch isolation technic on survival rates. Ann Surg 166:420-427

Umpleby HC, Williamson RC (1984) The efficacy of agents employed to prevent anastomotic recurrence in colorectal carcinoma. Ann R Coll Surg Engl 66:192-194

Umpleby HC, Williamson RC (1987) Anastomotic recurrence in large bowel cancer. Br J Surg 74:873-878

Umpleby HC, Fermor B, Symes MO, Williamson RC (1984) Viability of exfoliated colorectal carcinoma cells. Br J Surg 71:659-663

Umpleby HC, Ranson DL, Williamson RC (1985) Peculiarities of mucinous colorectal carcinoma. Br J Surg 72:715-718

Volpe C, Rodriguez Bigas M, Petrelli NJ (1996) Wide perineal dissection and its effect on local recurrence following potentially curative abdominoperineal resection for rectal adenocarcinoma. Cancer Invest 14:1-5

Westhues H (1934) Die pathologisch anatomischen Grundlagen der Chirurgie des Rektumkarzinoms. Thieme, Leipzig

Wiggers T, Jeekel J, Arends JW, Brinkhorst AP, Kluck HM, Luyk CI, Munting JD, Povel JA, Rutten AP, Volovics A (1988) No-touch isolation technique in colon cancer: a controlled prospective trial. Br J Surg 75:409–415

Willett CG, Compton CC, Shellito PC, Efird JT (1994) Selection factors for local excision or abdominoperineal resection of early stage rectal cancer. Cancer 73:2716–2720

Wimmenauer S, Keller H, Ruckauer KD, Rahner S, Wolff Vorbeck G, Kirste G, von Kleist S, Farthman EH (1997) Expression of CD44, ICAM-1 and N-CAM in colorectal cancer. Correlation with the tumor stage and the phenotypical characteristics of tumor-infiltrating lymphocytes. Anticancer Res 17:2395–2400

Zirngibl H, Husemann B, Hermanek P (1990) Intraoperative spillage of tumor cells in surgery for rectal cancer. Dis Colon Rectum 33:610–614

Radiochemotherapy as an Adjuvant Treatment for Rectal Cancer

L. Påhlman

Department of Surgery, University of Uppsala, Akademiska Sjukhuset, 75185 Uppsala, Sweden

Abstract

Adjuvant treatment with radiotherapy has been proposed in rectal cancer surgery, due to the high local recurrence rate. However, the rate varies substantially in the literature, an this may be one reason that adjuvant treatment is not obvious to all surgeons. The difference may be due to selection bias, different criteria for curative surgery, different follow-up routines, and/or the skill of the surgeon. The data are unequivocal from all randomized trials comparing surgery alone with surgery plus radiotherapy, given either pre- or postoperatively: the average local recurrence rate is about 29% in the surgery-alone arm. With pre- or postoperative radiotherapy the local recurrence rate is more or less halved. Moreover, preoperative irradiation is more dose efficient than postoperative irradiation, indicating that a higher dose must be used when postoperative radiotherapy is delivered, with an increased risk of damaging the normal surrounding tissues in the pelvis. This damage of normal tissue also has an impact on sphincter function and on postoperative small bowel obstruction. Since preoperative radiotherapy is more effective in killing tumor cells at a lower dose than postoperative treatment with or without chemotherapy, and since preoperative treatment is less toxic to normal tissues, preoperative radiotherapy should be used whenever radiotherapy for rectal cancer is considered.

Introduction

Rectal cancer is one of the most common malignant diseases in the western world. Even small benefits regarding survival will have an huge impact on overall survival and quality of life for this group of patients.

The rationale of combining surgery and radiotherapy with or without chemotherapy in this group of patients is obvious because of the different mechanisms of failure. Surgeons can only resect macroscopic disease such as tumour bulk, whereas radiotherapy can destroy micrometastases surrounding the tumour – areas not possible to excise during surgery without increased morbidity. The differences in local recurrence rates after surgery alone for resectable rectal cancer as reported in the literature (<5%–50%) really indicates that there is a need for better therapy, including better surgery. The difference between patient series reported in the literature in regard to both local recurrence rates and survival figures is probably an effect of patient selection, definitions of radicality and recurrence, the skill of the surgeon and follow-up procedures. However, in all reported randomized trials, the local recurrence rate in the surgery-alone arm exceeds 20% (average 28%), which actually shows the quality of standard rectal cancer surgery worldwide.

In order to improve treatment results, additional treatments such as radiotherapy, chemotherapy and immunotherapy have been tested. In regard to the use of adjuvant radiotherapy in resectable rectal cancer, no consensus has been achieved as to the optimal treatment in terms of dose levels and schedules, treatment time and timing. In this review, some aspects of radiobiology are presented. In particular, local recurrence rates and survival figures are discussed, as well as some aspects of adverse effects.

Dose Levels

For a probability of eradicating subclinical rectal cancer disease of more than 90%, a dose of at least 50 Gy using conventional fractionation is probably needed. These figures are based upon results obtained mainly from studies of breast and head-and-neck cancer (Fletcher 1984). It is fair to assume that the number of tumour cells to be killed by the radiotherapy is probably fewer before than after surgery, due to tumour cell proliferation and bad conditions for radiotherapy such as hypoxic tissues. On this assumption, the dose needs to be higher to reach the same efficacy if the treatment is given postoperatively than preoperatively.

In addition to depending on the total dose, the effect of radiation is also dependent upon the dose in each fraction and the total treatment time. In order to have a proper comparison between different trials regarding the biological effects of the various schedules, the radiation dose in this review has been estimated according to the linear-quadratic (LQ) formula, assuming that the α/β for the tumour is 10 Gy (Fowler 1989).

Local Recurrence Rates

It appears that the major cause of failure to cure pelvic tumours is lateral spread of microscopic tumour cells not removed at surgery (Ny et al. 1993; Adam et al. 1994). Since such a spread can reflect "bad" surgery, this may explain the difference in local recurrence rates seen in the literature. Moreover, these findings of microscopic lateral spread may also explain why radiotherapy reduces the recurrence rates. Table 1 presents data from all controlled randomized trials in which local recurrence rates have been reported.

Table 1. Pelvic recurrence after a combination of surgery and radiotherapy for rectal carcinoma (controlled trials with a surgery – alone group)

Reference	Irradiation		Surgery alone		Surgery + radiotherapy		Reduction (%)
	Dose (Gy)/number of fractions	LQ time	Number of local recurrences/total	%	Number of local recurrences/total	%	
Preoperative							
Goldberg et al. (1994)	15/3	22.5	51/210	24	31/185	17	29
Horn et al. (1990)	31.5	26.8	31/131	24	24/138	17	29
James et al. (1991)	20/4	30.0	58/141	41	26/143	18	56
Gérard et al. (1988)	34.5/15	35.2	49/175	28	24/166	14	50
MRC2[a] (MRC Trial Office 1996a)	40/20	36.0	50/132	38	41/129	32	16
Stockholm Rectal Cancer Study Group (1990)	25/5	37.5	120/485	28	61/424	14	50
Swedish Rectal Cancer Trial (1997)	25/5	37.5	150/557	27	63/553	11	58
Postoperative							
Balslev et al. (1986)	50/25	35.4	57/250	23	46/244	19	17
MRC3 (MRC Trial Office, 1996b)	40/20	36.0	69/235	29	43/234	20	31
Gastrointestinal Tumor Study Group (1985)	40–48/22	36.0	27/106	25	15/96	16	36
Fisher et al. (1988)	46.5/26	39.3	45/184	24	30/184	16	33
Arnaud et al. 1997	46/23	40.8	30/88	34	25/84	30	12
Treurniet-Donker et al. (1991)	50/25	43.8	28/84	33	21/88	24	27

LQ, Linear-quadratic formula.
[a] Tethered tumours only.

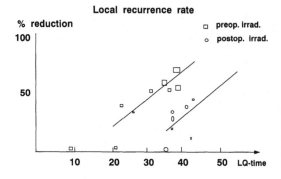

Fig. 1. Reductions in local recurrence rates in all controlled trials of adjuvant radiotherapy. Dose-response curves have been estimated for both preoperative and postoperative radiotherapy

In this table the reduction in local recurrence rate is given for each trial. It can be seen that the reductions in local recurrence rates are higher when radiotherapy is given preoperatively than postoperatively. Another interesting finding is that lower doses have generally been used in the trials using preoperative radiotherapy. This comparison thus further strongly supports the hypothesis that preoperative radiotherapy is more efficient than postoperative radiotherapy.

Figure 1 plots the reductions in local recurrence rates, expressed as percentages, against the radiation doses used in the same trials, distinguishing between preoperative and postoperative radiotherapy. A dose-response curve has been calculated for the preoperative trials. A dose-response curve cannot be calculated for the postoperative trials, but an estimated line has been drawn. These two dose-response curves show the difference in the doses used to attain the same goal. Postoperative irradiation doses must be at least 15 Gy higher to achieve the same reduction of local recurrence rates as preoperative radiation. Such high doses can be detrimental to the normal tissue surrounding the rectum.

Only one trial, the Uppsala trial in Sweden, has explicitly tested the question of whether or not preoperative radiotherapy is better than postoperative radiotherapy. This trial recruited 471 patients between 1980 and 1985. Patients with a Dukes' stage B or C tumour were randomly allocated to receive either preoperative radiotherapy (5×5.1 Gy in 1 week, LQ time = 38.0) followed by surgery the following week, or surgery followed by postoperative radiotherapy (60 Gy in 7–8 weeks, LQ time = 46.9). In the preoperative group the local recurrence rate was 12%, compared with 21% ($p<0.02$) in the postoperative group (Påhlman and Glimelius 1990). The dose used in the postoperative group is the highest dose ever given as an adjuvant treatment. Despite this, preoperative radiotherapy turned out to be better than postoperative radiotherapy. This trial thus also showed that the dose must be considerably higher if given postoperatively to reach the same efficacy a preoperatively administered dose, indicating that preoperative irradiation is the therapy of choice as an adjuvant treatment in rectal cancer surgery.

Effect on Survival

It is not likely that preoperative radiotherapy will have an impact on occult distant metastases, but with this treatment at moderate dose levels the reduction in local recurrence rate exceeds 50%. Since about 20% of patients with recurrent disease have local recurrence only, a slight effect on survival should be expected when preoperative radiotherapy is used. A meta-analysis of all controlled trials published up to 1984 showed a marginal positive effect of adjuvant irradiation, about 4%, on 5-year survival (Buyse et al. 1988).

Since this meta-analysis was published, several trials using higher doses have been published. In the preoperative EORTC trial, although the difference in survival does not reach statistical significance there is a tendency to better survival in the irradiated group of patients after prolonged follow-up (Gérard et al. 1988). A similar tendency to better cancer-specific survival was found in the two British trials, the Imperial Research Fund trial (Goldberg et al. 1994) and the North-West trial (James et al. 1991). In the Stockholm-Malmö trial, too, cancer specific survival was improved in the group of patients who received preoperative radiotherapy (Stockholm Rectal Cancer Study Group 1990). In a recent update of all patients in the Stockholm area, including some patients from the Swedish Rectal Cancer Trial, a statistically significant benefit of radiotherapy has been observed after a minimum follow-up of 3 years (Cedermark 1994). In the Swedish Rectal Cancer Trial 1168 patients were enrolled from 1987 to 1990. Patients were randomly allocated to surgery alone or preoperative (5×5 Gy in 1 week) radiotherapy (Swedish Rectal Cancer Trial 1996). Preliminary data after a minimum follow-up of 5 years shows statistically significantly better overall survival in the irradiated group of patients; 58% versus 48% (Swedish Rectal Cancer Trial 1997).

These good effects on cancer-specific or overall survival have not been found after postoperative radiotherapy alone. However, two trials have demonstrated a survival benefit when postoperative radiotherapy was combined with chemotherapy (5-FU and methyl-CCNU) (Gastrointestinal Tumor Study Group 1985; Fisher et al. 1988). Moreover, a third trial from the US has shown that chemotherapy in addition to radiotherapy improves survival (Krook et al. 1991). Since the effects on local recurrence rates in those trials were rather limited, and in one of the trials, a four-armed study (Gastrointestinal Tumor Study Group 1985), the survival figures with chemotherapy alone were almost the same as those in the combined treatment arm, it is tempting to believe that the survival benefit is an effect of the chemotherapy rather than of the postoperative radiotherapy.

Radiation Schedule

The rationale of using 5-Gy fractions instead of the more standardized 2-Gy fractions is a matter for discussion. Whatever dose per fraction used, it is important to reach a total dose equivalent to 40–50 Gy to have an effect on micrometastases. With conventional fractionation, i.e. 1.8-2.0 Gy daily, the patients have to be treated for 4.5 weeks. After this treatment surgery cannot be performed until 3-4 weeks later, giving a total preoperative treatment period of 2 months, which can be a troublesome period for both the patient and the surgeon. Moreover, the costs to society are high. The regimen of 5×5 Gy to a total dose of 25 Gy with surgery within the following week has been extensively used in Sweden (Påhlman and Glimelius 1990; Stockholm Rectal Cancer Study Group 1990, Swedish Rectal Cancer Trial 1996). This treatment schedule diminishes the interval from diagnosis to surgery substantially. However, the use of high-fraction doses is the cause of much concern since the risk of late adverse effects is theoretically higher, due to its decreased therapeutic ratio (see below).

Tolerance to Treatment

If radiotherapy is to be recommended, it is important that the treatment is well tolerated, i.e. that compliance is high. With preoperative irradiation compliance is more or less 100%. In the Uppsala trial only one patient assigned to preoperative radiotherapy did not receive the intended treatment because of refusal. In the postoperative radiotherapy group 84% of the patients started the treatment. Reasons for failure to receive treatment were in most cases postoperative complications or fatigue. The study design prescribes that the treatment should ideally start within 4-6 weeks after surgery, but only 50% of the patients started within 6 weeks and 24% did not start until after more than 2 months, usually due to problems with postoperative recovery (Påhlman et al. 1985). Similar difficulties were noted in the Danish trial (Balslev et al. 1986), where only 85% of the patients who started postoperative irradiation completed the treatment.

Acute Adverse Effects

Acute Toxicity

The short-term high-dose treatment used in Sweden is very well tolerated. Most patients have no discomfort. In one trial using 5-Gy fractions preoperatively, acute neurogenic pain of the lower lumbar region occurred immediately after irradiation in some patients (Påhlman and Glimelius 1990). In the entire experience in Uppsala since 1979, among the 550 patients who were treated with 5×5 Gy within prospective protocols, 32 reported pain. In only 6 patients (1%) did the pain persist for more than a few days, but 4 of these patients developed subacute neurogenic symptoms in a 6-month period, resulting in an inability to walk properly in 3 of them. The genesis of this potentially severe side effect is still unknown, but is probably due to some "hot" spots during radiotherapy, since it was more common in women than in men and occurred predominantly in obese patients with other diseases such as diabetes or previous neurologic disorders. Normally, higher doses than 5×5 Gy are required for nerves to be damaged by radiotherapy.

The acute toxicity from postoperative radiotherapy was also been prospectively studied in the Uppsala trial (Frykholm et al. 1993). Treatment was completed without any complications in only 9%, and in seven patients it was stopped. Although most patients were treated on an outpatient basis, five had to be hospitalized for parenteral nutrition due to diarrhoea. Fatigue, diarrhoea, skin reactions, urinary disorders and nausea occurred frequently in patients during the treatment period.

Postoperative Mortality

In two trials using preoperative radiotherapy, increased postoperative mortality has been reported among patients receiving irradiation (Stockholm Rectal Cancer Study Group 1990; Goldberg et al. 1994). The irradiation technique in those trials was 5-Gy fractions daily with two portals covering the whole pelvis and the abdominal cavity up to the mid L2 vertebra, giving a large part of the body the same dose as the tumour. The excess mortality was mainly noted in older patients (>75 years of age) and predominantly among those having generalized disease. The same radiation dose and schedule were also used in the Uppsala trial, but no increased postoperative mortality was found despite the each of any age restriction (Påhlman and Glimelius 1990). In the Uppsala trial a three-portal technique was used. In the recently published Swedish Rectal Cancer Trial (1993) no adverse effect on postoperative mortality was seen among the irradiated patients. Also in this trial the same high-dose radiotherapy (5×5 Gy within 1 week) but with the better three- or four-portal technique was used. When the irradiation is given using three or four portals, the volume of the body that receives the prescribed dose is much less than when using two portals, which probably explains the increased mortality figures seen after the two-portal technique was used. Since the causes of death among the patients in the two trials which reported increased postoperative mortality were mainly cardiovascular rather than infectious, it appears as if irradiation to a large body volume can be detrimental particularly to elderly patients.

Postoperative Morbidity

In the Swedish Rectal Cancer Trial 20% of the patients who underwent abdominal perineal excision and who received preoperative irradiation suffered perineal wound infection, compared with 10% in the non irradiated group (Swedish Rectal Cancer Trial 1993). This increase in perineal wound infections has been noticed in all trials using moderate- or high-dose preoperative radiotherapy (Påhlman and Glimelius 1990; Stockholm Rectal Cancer

Study Group 1990; Goldberg et al. 1994). This increase in perineal wound infection extended the hospital stay by approximately 2-3 days among the irradiated patients (Swedish Rectal Cancer Trial 1993). Other known complications after rectal cancer surgery, such as anastomotic dehiscence, deep vein thrombosis, urinary tract infections and abdominal wound infections, did not increase in incidence when preoperative radiotherapy was used.

Late Adverse Effects

Due to postoperative adhesions and the use of higher doses when postoperative radiotherapy is used, more late morbidity in the form of intestinal obstruction and/or diarrhoea would be expected among patients given postoperative irradiation than in those irradiated preoperatively, and this has in fact been reported (Frykholm et al. 1993; Mak et al. 1994). It looks as if the extent of this problem is related to the volume of small bowel included in the treatment volume (Letschert et al. 1990), and several techniques to reduce the amount of small bowel included within the irradiated volume have been proposed (Gallanger et al. 1986).

The Uppsala trial allowed preoperative irradiation (5×5 Gy in 1 week) to be compared with surgery alone as well as with postoperative radiotherapy, since in this trial the group of patients with Dukes' stage A tumours and allocated to postoperative radiotherapy had no radiotherapy. All patients with a follow-up period of 5-10 years have been reexamined with respect to late adverse effects of radiotherapy (Frykholm et al. 1993). There was no difference in cumulative risk of small bowel obstruction between the surgeryalone group and the preoperatively irradiated group (Frykholm et al. 1993). The risk in these two groups is just below 10%, compared with a 20% cumulative risk of having a small bowel obstruction after postoperative radiotherapy. These figures agree with other reports which show the incidence of small bowel obstruction to be up to 30%-40% if the beams extend high up in the abdomen (Balslev et al. 1986; Letschert et al. 1990). However, if the treatment is given with multiple pelvic fields, the risk of small bowel obstruction is decreased (Påhlman et al. 1985; Letschert et al. 1990).

Another concern with adjuvant radiotherapy is the risk of impaired sphincter function in the long term among patients who have undergone low anterior resection. In a report from a small series in the UK, it looks as though postoperative irradiation may have an adverse effect on sphincter function (Lewis et al. 1995). This phenomenon has also been observed in a small questionnaire study in the Uppsala material (Graf et al. 1996). Due to the small patient sample in both these reports it is not clear whether this is an adverse effect of irradiation. Theoretically, however, the irradiation might damage the sphincter or the pudendal nerve. A new questionnaire study among all patients enrolled in the Swedish Rectal Cancer Trial is in progress.

How Should We Use Radiotherapy Today?

The first step for surgeons facing patients with rectal cancer is to evaluate whether the tumour is mobile or not. If the tumour is not mobile, radiotherapy is more or less mandatory. In such cases the short preoperative treatment used extensively in Sweden is not the best option. However, if the tumour is considered mobile - meaning resectable and not fixed - adjuvant radiotherapy can be an option, since such treatment should be restricted to patients with a primarily resectable tumour. Of concern are patients with Dukes' stage A lesions, in whom radiotherapy probably is superfluous provided the surgery is optimized. These patients can easily be identified using endorectal ultrasound and withdrawn from adjuvant radiotherapy (Beyon et al. 1986).

Reports from Heald and Karanjia (1992), Enker et al. (1988) and Moriya et al. (1989) have shown that "optimized surgery" results in a very low frequency of local recurrences. Institutions with very low local recurrence rates can also be identified in the Swedish Rectal Cancer Trial. The magnitude of the decrease in the recurrence rates when preoperative irradiation was used is about the same (around 58%) among the "good" surgeons as for "bad" surgeons where the recurrence rates were high, indicating that recurrence can almost be eradicated if optimized surgery is combined with adjuvant radiotherapy.

It is important that radiotherapy be safe, both in the postoperative period and in the long term, since if radiotherapy is used in connection with optimized surgery, overtreatment is substantial. The experience from Uppsala since 1979 of using 25 Gy in 1 week combined with optimized surgical technique tells that the treatment is sufficiently safe (Påhlman and Glimelius 1990; Frykholm et al. 1993). However, experience at other institutions (Stockholm Rectal Cancer Study Group 1990), where the same dose was used but with a less optimal technique, shows that this treatment may be potentially hazardous.

The great discrepancy between the North American way of using adjuvant radiotherapy and the North European way is difficult to understand. In the United States, opinion is that all patients with a Dukes' B or C lesion should receive postoperative chemo- and radiotherapy (NCI, 1991). Based upon theoretical data and figures presented in all controlled randomized trials, there is no doubt that preoperative radiotherapy should be used - simply because it is more effective. As discussed above, the survival figures from the Swedish Rectal Cancer Trial are as good as those presented in the American trials. Moreover, the survival figures using postoperative combined radio- and chemotherapy are probably a chemotherapy effect. Therefore, the next step should be to combine preoperative radiotherapy with chemotherapy in the optimal way.

Treatment Policy in Uppsala Today

If a rectal tumour is assessed as non-resectable, i.e. fixed or not mobile, the patient is recommended to receive prolonged preoperative radiotherapy with 1.8-2 Gy fractions for a 4 to 5-week period. Whether chemotherapy should be added during the irradiation period in this group of patients is not known. To investigate this, a randomized trial is ongoing at our institution in which radiotherapy alone is compared with combined radio- and chemotherapy.

On the other hand, if the tumour is considered mobile, adjuvant treatment with 5×5 Gy is the option. Using preoperative endorectal ultrasound, tumours confined to the bowel wall are identified and excluded from radiotherapy, with one exception: if the tumour is situated very low in the lowest third of the rectum and abdominal perineal excision is the treatment option, preoperative irradiation is given, since that surgical procedure is tricky, especially in males. In all other patients where the endorectal examination shows tumour growth through the bowel wall, we advocate that preoperative radiotherapy (5×5 Gy) be used.

References

Adam IJ, Mohamdee MO, Martin EG et al (1994) Role of circumferential margin involvement in the local recurrence of rectal cancer. Lancet 344:707-711

Arnaud JP, Nordlinger B, Bosset JF, Boes GH, Shamoud T, Schlag PM, Rene F (1997) Radical surgery and postoperative radiotherapy as combined treatment in rectal cancer. Final results of a phase III study of European Organization for Research and Treatment of Cancer. Br J Surg 84:352-357

Balslev I, Pedersen M, Teglbjaerg PS et al (1986) Postoperative radiotherapy in Dukes B and C carcinoma of rectum and rectosigmoid. Cancer 58:22-28

Beynon J, Mortensen NJ McC, Foy DMA, Channer JL, Virjee J, Goddard P (1986) Preoperative assessment of local invasion in rectal cancer: digital examination, endoluminal sonography or computed tomography? Br J Surg 73:1015-1017

Buyse M, Zeleniuch-Jacquotte A, Chalmers TC (1988) Adjuvant therapy of colorectal cancer. Why we still don't know. JAMA 259:3571-3578

Cedermark B for the Stockholm Colo-rectal Study Group (1994) The Stockholm II trial on preoperative short term radiotherapy in operable rectal carcinoma. A prospective randomized trial. ASCO 13:577 (abstr)

Enker WE, Laffer UT, Block GE (1988) Enhanced survival of patients with colon and rectal cancer is based upon wide anatomical resection. Ann Surg 190:350-360

Fisher B, Wolmark N, Rockette H et al (1988) Postoperative adjuvant chemotherapy or radiation therapy for rectal cancer: results from NSABP Protocol R-01. J Natl Cancer Inst 80:21-29

Fletcher GH (1984) Subclinical disease. Cancer 53:1274-1284

Fowler JF (1989) The linear-quadratic formula and progress in fractionated radiotherapy. Br J Radiol 62:679-694

Frykholm G, Glimelius B, Påhlman L (1993) Pre- and postoperative irradiation in adenocarcinoma of the rectum: final treatment results of a randomized trial and an evaluation of late secondary effects. Dis Colon Rectum 36:564-572

Gallanger MJ, Brereton HD, Rostock RA et al (1986) A prospective study of treatment techniques to minimize the volume of pelvic small bowel with reduction of acute and late effects associated with pelvic irradiation. Int J Radiat Oncol Biol Phys 12:1565-1573

Gastrointestinal Tumor Study Group (1985) Prolongation of the disease-free interval in surgically treated rectal carcinoma. N Engl J Med 312:1464-1472

Gérard A, Buyse M, Nordlinger B et al (1988) Preoperative radiotherapy as adjuvant treatment in rectal cancer. Ann Surg 208:606-614

Goldberg PA, Nicholls RJ, Porter NH, Love S, Grimsey JF (1994) Long-term results of a randomized trial of short-course low-dose adjuvant pre-operative radiotherapy for rectal cancer: reduction in local treatment failure. Eur J Cancer 30A:1602-1606

Graf W, Ekström K, Glimelius B, Påhlman L (1996) Factors influencing bowel function after colorectal anastomosis. Dis Colon Rectum 39:744-749

Heald RJ, Karanjia ND (1992) Results of radical surgery for rectal surgery. World J Surg 16:848-857

Horn A, Halvorsen JF, Dahl O (1990) Preoperative radiotherapy in operable rectal cancer. Dis Colon Rectum 33:823-828

James RD, Haboubi N, Schofield PF, Mellor M, Salhab N (1991) Prognostic factors in colorectal carcinoma treated by preoperative radiotherapy and immediate surgery. Dis Colon Rectum 34:546-551

Krook JE, Moertel CG, Gunderson LL et al (1991) Effective surgical adjuvant therapy for high-risk rectal cancer. N Engl J Med 324: 709-715

Letschert JGJ, Lebesque JV, de Boer RW, Hart AAM, Bartelink H (1990) Dose-volume correlation in radiation-induced late small-bowel complications: a clinical study. Radiother Oncol 18:307-320

Lewis WG, Williamson MER, Kuzu A et al (1995) Potential disadvantages of postoperative adjuvant radiotherapy after anterior resection for rectal cancer: a pilot study of sphincter function, rectal capacity and clinical outcome. Int J Colorectal Disease 10:133-137

Mak AC, Rich TA, Schultheiss TE, Kavanagh B, Ota DM, Romsdahl MM (1994) Late complications of postoperative radiation for cancer of the rectum and rectosigmoid. Int J Radiat Oncol Biol Phys 28:597-603

Moriya Y, Hojo K, Sawada T et al (1989) Significance of lateral node dissection for advanced rectal carcinoma at or below the peritoneal reflection. Dis Colon Rectum 32:307-315

MRC Trial Office (1996a) Randomized trial of surgery alone versus radiotherapy followed by surgery for potentially operable encally advanced rectal cancer. Lancet 348:1605-1610

MRC Trial Office (1996b) Randomized trial of surgery alone versus surgery followed by radiotherapy for mobile cancer of the rectum. Lancet 348:1610-1614

NCI (1991) Clinical announcement. Adjuvant therapy for rectal cancer. National Cancer Institute, Bethesda, Md, 14 March

Ny IOL, Luk ISC, Yuen ST et al (1993) Surgical lateral clearance in resected rectal carcinomas; a multivariate analysis of clinicopathological features. Cancer 71:1972-1976

Påhlman L, Glimelius B (1990) Pre- and postoperative radiotherapy in rectal carcinoma: report from a randomized multicenter trial. Ann Surg 211:187-195

Påhlman L, Glimelius B, Graffman S (1985) Pre- versus postoperative radiotherapy in rectal carcinoma: an interim report from a randomized multicentre trial. Br J Surg 72:961-966

Stockholm Rectal Cancer Study Group (1990) Preoperative short-term radiation therapy in operable rectal carcinoma. A prospective randomized trial. Cancer 66:49-55

Swedish Rectal Cancer Trial (1993) Initial report from a Swedish multicentre study examining the role of preoperative irradiation in the treatment of patients with resectable rectal carcinoma. Br J Surg 80:1333-1336

Swedish Rectal Cancer Trial (1996) Local recurrence rate in a randomized multicentre trial of preoperative radiotherapy compared to surgery alone in resectable rectal carcinoma. Eur J Surg 162:397-402

Swedish Rectal Cancer Trial (1997) Improved survival with preoperative radiotherapy in resectable rectal cancer. N Engl J Med 336:980-987

Treurniet-Donker AD, van Putten WLJ, Wereldsma JCJ et al (1991) Postoperative radiation therapy for rectal cancer. Cancer 67:2042-2048

Intraoperative Radiotherapy as Adjuvant Treatment for Stage II/III Rectal Carcinoma

M. J. Eble[1], T. Lehnert[2], C. Herfarth[2], M. Wannenmacher[1]

[1] Department of Radiotherapy, Heidelberg University Hospital, Im Neuenheimer Feld 400, 69120 Heidelberg, Germany
[2] Department of Surgery, Heidelberg University Hospital, 69120 Heidelberg, Germany

Abstract

In recent years, many efforts have focused on combined radiotherapy and chemotherapy as adjuvants to curative surgery in patients with stage II and III (UICC) rectal carcinomas. Intraoperative radiotherapy (IORT) makes it possible to increase the total irradiation dose in a locally restricted area while sparing normal mobile organs, but it is limited by increased late toxicity. A prospective phase I/II study was designed to evaluate the efficacy of moderate-dose intraoperative and external beam radiotherapy (IO-EBRT), in some cases with concomitant chemotherapy.

Sixty-three patients with a stage II or III rectal carcinoma were eligible for analysis (median follow-up 30.6 months). Fifty-four patients had undergone a complete resection (R0). Mean IORT dose was 11.3 Gy and mean EBRT dose 41.4 Gy. In 45 patients (71.4%) concomitant chemotherapy was delivered (5-FU, leucovorin).

Two patients suffered local failure. However, overall local tumor control was markedly improved compared to historical controls (96.8% vs 66.2%). Patients treated with IO-EBRT showed a reduced incidence of distant metastases after concomitant chemotherapy (17.6% vs 38.8%). A 4-year actuarial relapse-free survival of 82% was obtained after IO-EBRT plus chemotherapy, and 59% after IO-EBRT alone. The postoperative course was unremarkable in 47.6% of patients. No radiation colitis or neuropathy occurred.

Moderate-dose IORT and EBRT is safe, taking into account related late toxicities. It is an effective local treatment approach, resulting in an encouraging local control rate.

Introduction

Regrowth of cancer of the rectum after apparently complete resection is common. Local recurrence correlates to prognosis, i.e. survival, after surgical resection alone. These recurrences are rarely curable, and in addition are often difficult to treat palliatively. In recent years extensive consideration has been given to using radiotherapy and chemotherapy as adjuvants to "curative" surgery in patients with tumors penetrating through the full thickness of the rectal wall or metastasizing to regional lymph nodes (stages II and III according to the UICC staging system). The 1990 National Institutes of Health Consensus Development Conference Panel recommended combined postoperative chemotherapy and radiation therapy for patients with stage II and stage III rectal carcinoma (NIH Consensus Conference 1990). The panel concluded that, at that time, the most effective regimen appeared to be 5-FU chemotherapy and high-dose pelvic irradiation.

The minimum effective dose to improve local tumor control has not been established, but at least 50 Gy over 5 weeks is recommended. Late severe colitis rates increase dramatically with doses of more than 45 Gy. Postoperative small bowel obstruction after surgery alone can occur in up to 6% of patients (Gunderson et al. 1985; Saxton et al. 1982), but the risk may rise to as high as 25%–37% with the addition of postoperative large field irradiation (Letschert et al. 1990; Vigliotti et al. 1987). The risk of small bowel obstruction is related to the volume irradiated; with the use of modern irradiation techniques this risk has been reduced to 5%–9% (Eble et al. 1995; Mak et al. 1994).

Intraoperative radiotherapy is limited as to dose by an increased risk of late adverse effects. In a study at the Mayo Clinic neuropathies were observed in 32% of the patients after intraoperative radiotherapy with a median dose of 17.5 Gy added to an external beam dose of 50.4 Gy (Shaw et al. 1990). A phase I/II study was initiated at the University of Heidelberg in June 1991 in which patients received a moderate dose of external beam radiotherapy (<45 Gy) either before or after surgery combined with a moderate-dose intraoperative electron beam boost (10–15 Gy). During the early part of this pilot study a combined-modality approach using concomitant chemotherapy was established.

Patients and Methods

Patients

Between June 1991 and December 1994, 104 patients with clinically advanced cT3, T4, or N+ tumors (stages II, III, UICC classification) were treated with intraoperative radiotherapy (IORT). Patients were selected for IORT on the basis of endoscopic ultrasound examination and computed tomography of the pelvis in patients suffering from tumor-related stenosis. Initial assessment included an additional clinical examination, chest X-ray, proctoscopy, colonoscopy, and serum chemical analysis. Twenty-two patients were found to be ineligible for analysis of local control and survival; these patients either had distant metastases ($n=12$) at the time of surgery, a stage I rectal carcinoma ($n=17$), or macroscopic residual disease ($n=1$), or else refused external beam radiotherapy ($n=8$). One patient died postoperatively, one patient proved to have a secondary carcinoma, and one patient was lost to follow-up 15 months after IORT. The mean age of the remaining 63 patients was 56.6 years. Surgical procedures were anterior resection in 34 patients, abdominoperineal resection in 28, and a Hartmann procedure in 1 patient. The distal, proximal, and radial margins of all surgical specimens were assessed. Radial margins were microscopically positive for disease in 9 patients (14.3%).

The efficacy of IO-EBRT with concomitant chemotherapy and without it was compared to results in a historical control group treated at our institution with EBRT alone. There were no significant differences in external beam irradiation technique – i.e., target volume definition, beam energy, and dose prescription – nor in patient-related prognostic factors – i.e., patient age and sex distribution – nor in tumor-related prognostic factors – i.e., stage distribution and tumor location – between the study group and the historical control group (Table 1).

Intraoperative Radiotherapy

IORT started in the Department of Surgery in June 1991 with a dedicated facility installed in the central operating theater. A magnetron-powered linear accelerator (Siemens Mevatron ME) provides electron beam energies ranging

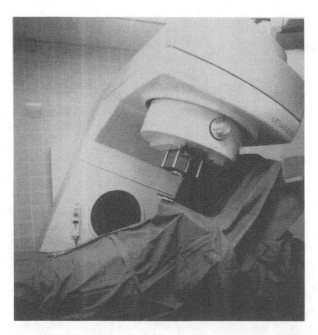

Fig. 1. Dedicated linear accelerator for intraoperative radiotherapy (IORT) installed in the central operating theater. The gantry is mounted on the wall of the operation room, which allows application of the electron beam at different angles

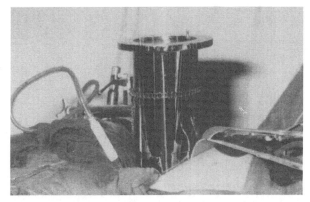

Fig. 2. Beam collimation within the patient was achieved with circular applicators. Different applicator sizes allowed appropriate delineation of the target volume

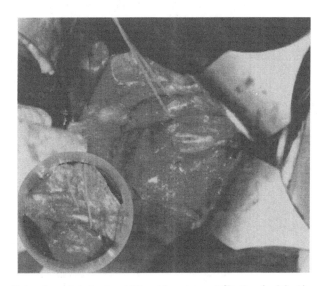

Fig. 3. A 47-year old patient suffering from clinically staged T4 rectal carcinoma infiltrating the left side wall of the pelvis. After tumor resection electron beam IORT was given. The *inset* shows a view through the applicator

from 6 to 18 MeV, corresponding to a treatment depth of 20–54 mm (90% isodose) (Fig. 1). The beam was collimated with round beveled (22°) chrome-plated brass applicators. Applicator diameters varied from 6 to 9 cm (6 cm, $n=14$; 8 cm, $n=43$; 9 cm, $n=6$) (Fig. 2). The beam was aligned using an "air docking" procedure, guided by an arrangement of four pairs of laser beams emerging from the gantry. Each pair intersected to form one of four points every 90° along a 152-mm-diameter circle on an alignment plate placed on the applicator entrance. Precise alignment was obtained with a modified operation table trolley, providing fine adjustment in all three axes.

As reported elsewhere (Eble et al. 1994), in most patients with a nontethered rectal carcinoma (clinically staged as T3) IORT target volume included the presacral/precoccygeal area and the lower part of both pelvic side walls. After resection of a tumor attached to the pelvic side wall, that side wall was included in its entirety (Fig. 3). In two patients with a carcinoma fixed to the prostate, the posterior part of the prostate was irradiated separately. Electron beam IORT was prescribed to the 90% isodose and delivered at a dose rate of 9 Gy/min. Mean IORT dose was 11.3 Gy (range 10–15 Gy).

External Beam Radiotherapy and Chemotherapy

External beam radiotherapy (EBRT) was delivered with 23-MV photons. A three-field technique (equally weighted posterior and lateral fields) was used with the cephalad field borders at L4–L5 and the inferior borders 4–5 cm distal to the tumor. The lateral borders of the posteroanterior field were 1 cm outside the true bony pelvis. The perineal scar after abdominoperineal resection was included in the target volume. The posterior border of the lateral fields was 1 cm behind the flat surface of the sacrum. The patient lay prone on an open table top device. Mean EBRT dose was 41.1±1.4 Gy, determined to the reference point, according to ICRU 50. Doses were delivered at a conventional fractionation of 1.8 Gy/fraction, 5 fractions/week. Three-dimensional treatment planning was carried out for all patients on the basis of continuous CT slices of 1 cm thickness. Eight patients underwent preoperative radio- or radiochemotherapy ($n=6$). Surgery was performed 35.8±8.4 days thereafter. Forty-five patients received concomitant intravenous chemotherapy, which consisted of bolus intravenous leucovorin (200 mg/m^2 per hour) and intravenous bolus fluorouracil (400 mg/m^2 per hour) on days 1–5 and 22–26 of the EBRT, followed by another 4 weekly cycles (each cycle after 2 weeks rest).

Results

Morbidity

Surgical morbidity was similar to that seen in historical controls. None of the patients died from complications of treatment. The risk of perineal wound dehiscence after abdominoperineal resection and primary wound closure ($n=27$), including even small and superficial lesions, was 18.5% ($n=5$). Two of these patients had preoperative EBRT. In the remaining 3 patients EBRT started 32–67 days after surgery. Pelvic abscesses were observed in 5 patients (7.9%). Fistula formation at the anastomosis occurred in 6 patients who had undergone anterior resection ($n=34$) (17.6%). Disturbance of micturition was noted in 17 patients (27%). Other perioperative complications included a deep thrombosis of the leg in 1 patient, a secondary hemorrhage in 1 patient, and herniation of the small bowel requiring surgical revision in 1 patient. Counting all perioperative complications, major and minor, at least 30 patients remained (47.6%) who had an unremarkable perioperative course.

Local Control and Patient Survival

The median follow-up in the 63 evaluable patients was 30.6 months. Eighteen patients had intraoperative and external beam radiotherapy (IO-EBRT) alone while 45 patients had concomitant chemotherapy in addition. To describe the effect of dose escalation, patients in the historical control group were stratified according to the total radiation dose given, giving the following historic subgroups: moderate-dose EBRT (46–51 Gy), 27 patients; high-dose EBRT (52–66 Gy), 38 patients. Patients with moderate-dose EBRT had a median follow-up of 33.4 months and those with high-dose EBRT a median follow-up of 37.6 months.

Local tumor control was markedly improved after IO-EBRT. Two of 45 patients (95.5%) treated with IO-EBRT and concomitant chemotherapy suffered infield recurrence 18.3 and 21.9 months afterwards respectively. At the time of primary treatment both had a locally advanced stage III rectal carcinoma (pT3 N3 M0 L1, pT4 N3 M0 L1, respectively). Local tumor control was achieved in 100% of patients treated with IO-EBRT alone. Microscopically incomplete resection had no impact on local control. Twenty-two patients (33.8%) of the control group, treated with EBRT alone, suffered locally recurrence within the pelvis. The median relapse-free interval was 10.5 months. Increased radiation doses yielded a marked improvement in local tumor control (55.6% with $\leqslant 52$ GY v 73.7% with $\geqslant 52$ Gy).

Table 1. Comparative data for the study group and historical controls. Figures are given as percentages

	Study group		Historical controls	
	IO-EBRT + chemotherapy ($n=45$)	IO-EBRT ($n=18$)	EBRT ≤ 51 GY ($n=27$)	EBRT ≥ 52 GY ($n=38$)
TNM stage				
T2 N+	4.4	5.5	18.6	7.9
T3 N0	33.3	38.9	11.1	31.6
T3 N+	40.0	33.4	62.9	34.1
T4 N0	13.4	5.5	3.7	18.4
T4 N+	8.9	16.7	3.7	7.9
Stage III (UICC)	53.4	55.5	85.2	50.1
R0	84.4	88.8	92.6	81.6
Preoperative radiotherapy	13.3	11.1	0	13.1

R0, Resection without macroscopically or microscopically detectable residual disease

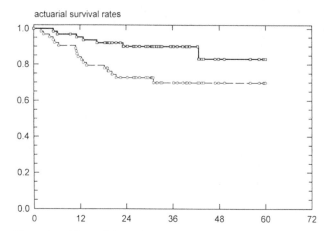

Fig. 4. Actuarial overall *(squares)* and relapse-free survival *(circles)* in 63 patients treated with intraoperative and external beam radiotherapy

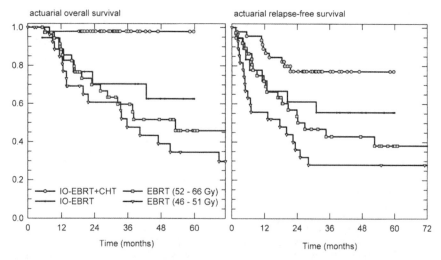

Fig. 5. Actuarial overall *(left)* and relapse-free survival *(right)* in patients with a stage II or III rectal carcinoma. Results are shown in relation to total dose given in external beam radiotherapy, additional IORT, and concomitant chemotherapy (IO-EBRT + CHT)

The distant metastasis rate was improved by adding chemotherapy (17.6% vs 38.8%). No difference was observed between controls (35% with >52 Gy, 40% with <51 Gy) and the subgroup of patients who had IO-EBRT without chemotherapy. The 4-year actuarial overall survival rate for all 63 patients was 82%, while relapse-free survival for the same period was 70% (Fig. 4). Both the improved local control from IORT and the reduced distant metasta-

Table 2. Results in the study group and the historical controls

	Local control (%)	Distant metastases (%)
IO-EBRT + chemotherapy ($n=45$)	95.6	17.8
IO-EBRT ($n=18$)	100	38.8
EBRT ≥52 Gy ($n=38$)	72.3	36.2
EBRT ≤51 Gy ($n=27$)	55.6	40.7

sis rate from concomitant chemotherapy had an impact on relapse-free survival (Fig. 5; Table 2).

Discussion

Intraoperative boost irradiation of residual disease after resection of rectal carcinoma has been shown to be efficacious in a few institutional trials. Results from the Mayo Clinic, using a combined approach of surgical resection with IORT (15-20 Gy) after high-dose EBRT (50.4 Gy) have been recently published (Gunderson et al. 1997). In that series, all patients suffered from a locally advanced, initially unresectable primary tumor of the colon or rectum. Thirty-nine of 56 patients underwent concomitant chemotherapy. Overall local control was 87%, which was not significantly improved after additional chemotherapy. Forty-eight percent of patients developed distant metastases, but the figure was significantly reduced in patients who had combined chemo-radiotherapy (36% vs 77%, $p=0.013$). As a consequence, 5-year overall and relapse-free survival was significantly improved with the combined treatment approach (54% vs 9%, $p=0.01$). A relationship between IORT dose and incidence of grade 2 or 3 neuropathy was observed (<12.5 Gy, 3% grade 2 or 3 neuropathy; >15 Gy, 23%; $p=0.03$).

At the M.D. Anderson Cancer Center patients with locally advanced primary rectal carcinomas had preoperative radiotherapy (45 Gy) combined with protracted continuous infusion of 5-fluorouracil (Weinstein et al. 1995). Selected patients with adherent tumors at surgery received intraoperative boost irradiation. Eleven of 37 patients thus had IO-EBRT. In this group of patients a higher percentage of tumors penetrated the bowel wall (100% vs 50%) or had close or positive resection margins (55% vs 19%). While the incidence of distant metastasis in that subgroup was markedly increased (64% vs 19%), local control was as high as in the group without IORT (100% vs, 96%).

In our phase I/II study IORT was implemented as a boost technique in an adjuvant treatment regimen. IORT was given to all patients who revealed a stage II or III rectal carcinoma on endoscopic ultrasonography. The benefit expected from this technique was twofold: in addition to the anticancer effect, during IORT maximum sparing of the small bowel was possible by simply retaining it out of the target volume. With modern EBRT techniques, including three-dimensional treatment planning, the dose was limited to 41.4 Gy, in view of the tolerance level for late small bowel sequelae. If radiation therapy is to be an effective local treatment technique for rectal carcinomas, high or moderately high radiation doses will be necessary. IORT allows locally restricted dose escalation, but from previous data the IORT dose should be limited to less than 15 Gy to avoid late adverse effects, e.g. neuropathy. None of our patients complained of neuropathy or small bowel obstruction, except the one who suffered herniation of the small bowel postoperatively. On the basis of our data we can conclude that this multi-modality approach using moderate-dose IORT (10-12 Gy) and moderate-dose EBRT (41.4 Gy) is feasible, safe, and results in very low local recurrence rates, even in patients with microscopic residual disease or close resection margins. Furthermore, the combined chemo-radiation approach reduced the risk of developing distant metastases and thus improved survival.

References

Eble MJ, Kallinowski F, Wannenmacher M, Herfarth C (1994) Intraoperative Radiotherapie des lokal ausgedehnten und rezidivierten Rektumkarzinoms. Chirurg 65:585-592

Eble MJ, Wulf J, Kampen M, Weischedel U, Wannenmacher M (1995) Lokal begrenzte Dosiseskalation in der Radiotherapie des primär ausgedehnten und lokal rezidivierten Rektumkarzinoms. Strahlenther Onkol 171:77-86

Gunderson LL, Russell AH, Lewellyn HJ, Doppke KP, Tepper JE (1985) Treatment planning for colorectal cancer: radiation and surgical techniques and value of small-bowel films. Int J Radiat Oncol Biol Phys 11:1379-1393

Gunderson LL, Nelson H, Martenson JA, Cha S, Haddock M, Devine R, Fiedck JM, Wolff B, Dozois R, O'Conell MJ (1997) Locally advanced primary colorectal cancer: intraoperative electron and external beam irradiation +/-5-FU. Int J Radiat Oncol Biol Phys 37:601-614

Letschert JGJ, Lebesque JV, de Boer RW, Hart AAM, Bartelink H (1990) Dose-volume correlation in radiation-related small bowel complications: a clinical study. Radiother Oncol 18:307-320

Mak A, Rich TA, Schultheiss TE, Kavanagh B, Ota DM, Romsdahl MM (1994) Late complications of postoperative radiation therapy for cancer of the rectum and rectosigmoid. Int J Radiat Oncol Biol Phys 28:597-603

NIH Consensus Conference (1990) Adjuvant therapy for patients with colon and rectal cancer. JAMA 1264:1444-1450

Saxton JP, Withers HR, Romsdahl MM, Borgelt BB (1982) The use of irradiation therapy in the treatment of tumors of the rectum of rectosigmoid. J Natl Med Assoc 74:529-533

Shaw EG, Gunderson LL, Martin JK (1990) Peripheral nerve and ureteral tolerance of intraoperative radiation therapy: clinical and dose response analysis. Radiother Oncol 18:247-261

Vigliotti A, Rich TA, Romsdahl MM, Withers HR, Oswald MJ (1987) Postoperative adjuvant radiotherapy for adenocarcinoma of the rectum and rectosigmoid. Int J Radiat Oncol Biol Phys 13:999-1006

Weinstein GD, Rich TA, Shumate CR, Skibber JM, Clearly KR, Ajani JA, Ota DM (1995) Preoperative infusional chemoradiation and surgery with or without an electron beam intraoperative boost for advanced primary rectal cancer. Int J Radiat Oncol Biol Phys 32:197-204

Radical Sphincter Preservation Surgery with Coloanal Anastomosis Following High-Dose External Irradiation for the Very Low Lying Rectal Cancer

G. J. Marks[1], J. H. Marks[1], M. Mohiuddin[2], and L. Brady[3]

[1] Comprehensive Rectal Cancer Center, Department of Surgery, Allegheny University of the Health Sciences, Broad and Vine, Mail Stop 413, Philadelphia, PA 19102-1192, USA
[2] Department of Radiation Oncology, University of Kentucky, Lexington, Kentucky, USA
[3] Comprehensive Rectal Cancer Center, Department of Radiation Oncology and Nuclear Medicine, Allegheny University of the Health Sciences, Philadelphia, Pennsylvania, USA

Abstract

High-dose preoperative radiation and specifically designed surgical techniques were used to extend the application of sphincter preservation surgery for cancer of the distal 3 cm of the true rectum. A total of 203 consecutive patients with rectal cancer were treated with external-beam irradiation (45–70 Gy) and radical curative surgery. The cancer was at the level of 0.5–3.0 cm in 65 patients. In these 65 patients treated by radical resection with coloanal anastomosis six suffered recurrence (9%), and the 5-year actuarial survival was 85%. There was a single death. There was no local recurrence among 44 patients in whom the postradiated cancer resided in the rectal wall with or without nodal involvement. With proper selection, high-dose preoperative radiation therapy thus permits extended use of sphincter preservation surgery with coloanal anastomosis for cancers of the distal 3 cm of the true rectum.

Introduction

Quality of life issues have assumed a dominant role in the management of the rectal cancer patient. The high risk of locoregional recurrence and the frequent loss of anal sphincter function present the greatest threats to quality of life. These issues are targeted by the use of preoperative high-dose external irradiation, which has gained recognition for its ability to down-stage the rectal cancer and, theoretically, to sterilize the regional microlymphatics (Marks et al. 1992). These effects have brought a reduction in locoregional recurrence and, in non-randomized studies, improved survival following multimodal rectal cancer surgery (Mendenhall et al. 1985).

We have reasoned that the ability of high-dose preoperative external irradiation to down-stage and sterilize the microlymphatics allows smaller circumferential and distal margins to be safely used in accomplishing sphincter preservation surgery for the low lying rectal cancer. We are treating patients with select cancers of the distal rectum between the 0.5-cm and 3-cm level superior to the anorectal ring by surgical sphincter preservation after high-dose irradiation, and our experience with these patients provides the subject of this report.

Following high-dose external irradiation, cancers of the distal 3 cm of the rectum that are mobile 5.5–8 weeks after radiation are operated upon by an original technique of transanal abdominal transanal radical proctosigmoidectomy and descending coloanal anastomosis (TATA). The observed low rate of locoregional recurrence and the improved survival in this subset of patients suggests a true quality-of-life benefit from this multi-modality program.

Experiences with high-dose preoperative irradiation for fixed and inoperable rectal cancer dating to the early 1960s and subsequent experience with the surgical reconstruction of the radiation-necrotic rectum were the background for the development of a program, initiated in 1976, of high-dose preoperative irradiation and sphincter preservation surgery for unfavorable and distal rectal cancer. With the confidence drawn from having performed an anastomosis in the distal 2 cm of a radiation-injured rectum, it was posited that by following the same surgical principles, an anastomosis could be safely accomplished after irradiating cancers at the greatest risk for local failure, i.e., prospectively staged unfavorable or low lying rectal cancers (Marks 1973, 1976).

Initially, the combined abdominotranssacral method was used exclusively to accomplish sphincter preservation (Marks et al. 1985). Presuming a need for a 2- or 3-cm margin distal to the cancer, sphincter preservation was originally limited to those tumors at and above the 4 cm level relative to the anorectal ring. As data accumulated revealing a local recurrence rate between 10% and 12%, centimeter by centimeter, cancers lower in the rectum were treated with restorative surgery. In 1984, a new surgical technique was designed to allow safe resection of tumors below the 2-cm level. We called this procedure the transanal abdominal transanal radical proctosigmoidectomy with direct coloanal anastomosis (TATA), and its uniqueness is in the initiating of the mobilization of the rectum transanally. It has become the standard technique used for all mobile cancers in the distal 3 cm of the rectum. The benefit of this method derives from beginning the dissection of the distal rectum by the transanal route, which assures a maximal and known distal margin to the cancer and avoids the pitfall of not being able, through an abdominal approach, to palpate a previously irradiated small, very low lying rectal cancer. This method also obviates the need to apply a clamp distal to the tumor in what is frequently an uncomfortably narrow and confined space. We present here data relative to the first consecutive 65 patients with cancer in the distal 3 cm of the rectum who were treated with transanal abdominal transanal radical proctosigmoidectomy with coloanal anastomosis (TATA) after high-dose external irradiation.

Methods

Since 1976, all patients seen in the Comprehensive Rectal Cancer Center with biopsy-proven invasive rectal cancer, exclusive of those cancers suited for local excision and those assessed to be confined to the rectal wall at or above the 7-cm level, were selected for high-dose preoperative external irradiation after joint evaluation by both the surgeon and the radiation oncologist. Details of tumor assessment were recorded as follows: level in the rectum relative to the anorectal ring; site on the wall; size; configuration; depth of ulceration; percentage of circumference involved; degree of fixation; absence or presence of obstruction; palpability of lymph nodes; and prospective stage. Prospective staging was augmented by endorectal sonography, CT scan, and more recently, rectal coil MRI unless interdicted by local factors. After prospectively staging of the cancer clinically, all patients with favorable rectal cancers at or above the 7-cm level, where sphincter preservation is not in doubt, were assigned to the selective sandwich program that employs a single treatment of 500 cGy immediately prior to any suitable sphincter preservation surgery. Those patients with tumors proved histologically to be T3 or N-positive were treated with postoperative radiation. All other patients (i.e., those with unfavorable cancers at any level or those with favorable cancers at or below the 6-cm level) were treated preoperatively with 4500–7000 cGy in fractions of 180–250 cGy over a period of 4.5–7 weeks. The appreciation of dose-related benefits has brought us to select 5580 cGy in 180-cGy fractions as the customary dose (Ahmad et al. 1993). A post-radiation interval of 4.5–8 weeks preceded surgery. Selection for sphincter preservation has evolved to include all patients with cancers from the 0.5-cm level upward, except where the cancer at or below the 3-cm level remained fixed after irradiation.

Radiation Treatment Parameters

Radiation is delivered using high-energy photons ($\geq$10-MeV). A minimal tumor dose of 4500 cGy over 5 weeks at 180 cGy per fraction (or an equivalent dose of 4000 cGy at 250 cGy per fraction) is delivered to the whole pelvis. A four-field box technique with shaped anteroposterior/postanterior and lateral fields is used. The superior border is at the L5–S1 junction with the perineum and anal canal included inferiorly. The lateral borders extend 1 cm beyond the bony pelvis. The posterior border encompasses the whole of the sacrum with adequate margins and lateral fields to include all external and internal iliac lymph nodes. All fields are treated daily, 5 days a week. Patients with tumor fixation are given an additional boost of 1000–1500 cGy using a reduced field that encompasses the tumor and presacral tissues.

Operative Technique

The anesthetized patient is placed in a supine lithotomy position with the lower extremities in Allen stirrups and care taken to protect the common peroneal nerve. Digital rectal examination is performed to confirm the site and characteristics of the tumor – information that may be advantageous in planning the dissection strategy. Two Betadine-soaked 4×4 gauze sponges are tied together and inserted into the rectum. The skin of the abdomen and perineum are surgically prepared and draped in continuity. The vagina is always prepared. With the buttocks extending over the edge of the table and the patient in an exaggerated lithotomy position, epinephrine solution 1-200 000 concentration is infiltrated into the posterior, lateral, and anterior perirectal tissue, avoiding penetration of the needle into the rectum. Allis-

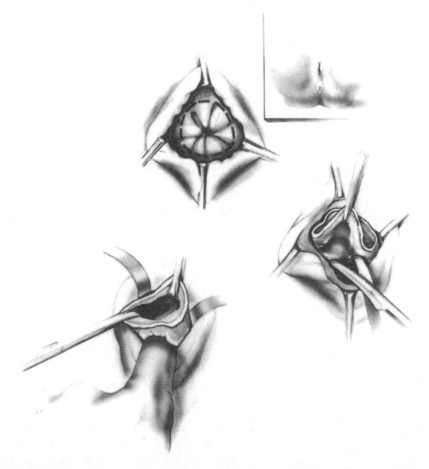

Fig. 1. With the patient in the exaggerated lithotomy position, transanal dissection is begun by full-thickness incision through the anorectal wall at or immediately above the pectinate line

Adair clamps are used to stoutly grasp the anal canal and bring about its gentle eversion.

The exposed anal canal is washed with Betadine. Epinephrine solution is injected submucosally and intramurally. The mucosa is incised circumferentially with the electrocautery at a point 3 to 7 mm superior to the pectinate line, allowing for a maximal distal margin (Fig. 1). Scissors introduced into the posterior midline are spread to permit penetration through the full thickness of the anorectal wall to reach the interval between the wall and puborectalis muscle (Fig. 2). A lighted suction device aids in visualizing the whitish adventitial surface of the puborectalis muscle, which marks the proper plane, the key to successful dissection. Blunt dissection enlarges the plane in both lateral directions (Fig. 3). The incision through the full thickness of the wall must be extended circumferentially and completely to avoid a shearing effect when the pressure of finger dissection develops. Completion of the incision through mucosa and muscle anteriorly requires special care because redundant mucosa tends to obscure non-incised segments of mucosa and wall. Failure to recognize an incomplete incision confounds the anterior extrarectal dissection. The transected end of the rectum is grasped sequentially with Allis-Adair clamps for proper traction, and extra care is taken when the tumor is very low lying.

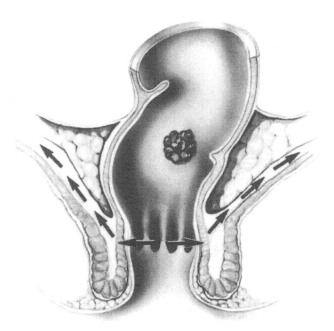

Fig. 2. Dissection is carried out in the interval between the internal sphincter muscles and the puborectalis. The external sphincter, puborectalis, and levator ani muscles are not disturbed, and one or two centimeters of internal sphincter is preserved

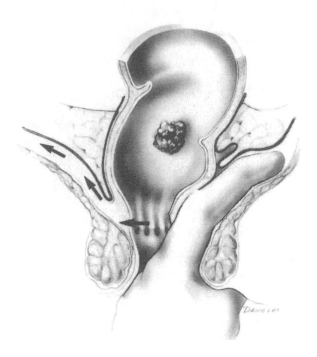

Fig. 3. Once established, the plane of dissection is enlarged by blunt fingertip dissection

Blunt and sharp extrarectal dissection is pursued first in the posterior region where landmarks are more readily appreciated. It is important not to stray deep or lateral to the puborectalis or the levator ani muscles. The coccyx and the anterior sacrococcygeal ligament are helpful palpable landmarks. The yellow fat that surrounds the rectum is a visual guide. A sweeping motion with the finger frees the perirectal tissue laterally and usually strips the endopelvic fascia, which becomes an additional protective tissue barrier for the rectum and its contained cancer and mesorectum. The need to avoid dissection deep to the levator ani muscle is ever present. In the male patient, palpably locating the capsule of the prostate anteriorly and using that as a guide for the development of the proper anterior plane is critical. Avoidance of the urethra is aided by this maneuver, as is dissection in the lateral paraprostatic sulcus, a common pitfall. Anterior application of narrow retractors with posterior displacement of the rectum permits appreciation of the arching fibers of the puborectalis muscle, which upon transection is one of the few places active bleeding may occur. Such bleeding is easily managed with electrocoagulation. Blunt dissection concludes in the region of the seminal vesicles or at the level of the cervix. The transected end of the rectum is then closed with an inverting watertight suture. The pelvis is thoroughly la-

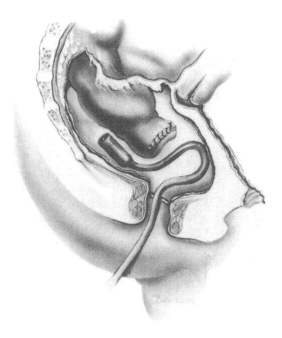

Fig. 4. The rectum is mobilized circumferentially to the level of the cervix or seminal vesicles. The open end of the rectum is closed with an inverting continuous running suture, and a red rubber catheter is placed in the pelvis and fixed perianally

vaged with topical kanamycin solution and the pelvis inspected for bleeding. The open end of a #24 red rubber catheter is inserted into the pelvis and fixed externally with a perianal suture (Fig. 4). A series of sterile towels cover the perineum and secure the electocautery probe and suction device for reclaiming during the final perineal phase.

The patient's legs are lowered to 15° flexion, and there is an exchange of instruments, gloves, and gowns, following which the previously prepared and sterile abdomen is addressed by a generous midline or left rectus incision from the symphysis to the xiphoid. Intraperitoneal exploration is carried out with selective intraoperative hepatic sonography. The sigmoidocolic junction is marked with a black silk suture prior to incising the lateral peritoneal reflection of the sigmoid and left colon. The left colon is mobilized and the splenic flexure released by blunt and sharp retroperitoneal dissection. The omentum is freed to the midpoint of the transverse colon. Upon total release of the splenic flexure, the colorenal ligament is incised and the fusion plane between the retroperitoneum and the mesocolon identified. Proceeding along the fusion plane, the retroperitoneum is displaced posteriorly and the mesocolon is brought medially. The ureter is usually identified without difficulty, but if it is not, it can be found as it crosses the external iliac artery approximately 1 cm lateral to the origin of the hypogastric artery. Once identified, it is gently displaced posteriorly through its course. The lateral peritoneal reflection of the sigmoid colon is incised, and the incision is continued into the pelvis pararectally to the cul de sac. The posterior parietal peritoneum to the right of the aorta is incised just inferior to the duodenojejunal junction, and the incision is carried distally over the brim of the pelvis in a pararectal position to the cul de sac, where it is brought anteriorly to meet its counterpart. The distal sigmoid colon is encircled with a stout cloth to prevent the sponges that have been introduced into the rectum from migrating proximally. The sigmoid colon is held taut anteriorly to aid in visualizing the hypogastric nerve plexus, which is displaced posteriorly and opens the plane for the posterior mobilization of the rectum. Once accomplished, the dissection is carried laterally in a generally bloodless plane. The lateral stalks with the middle hemorrhoidal vessels occupying a more medial position than customary are identified, transected, and secured.

Mobilization of the rectum is remarkably simplified because of the initial transanal stage. The rectum is delivered from the pelvis and covered with an

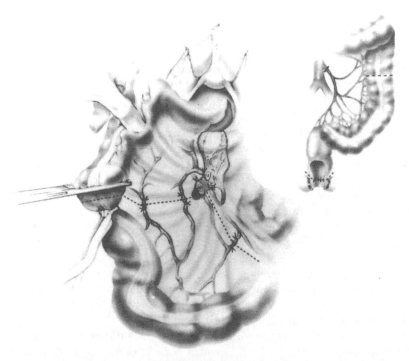

Fig. 5. Following repositioning, proctosigmoidectomy is carried out transabdominally with high ligation of the inferior mesenteric pedicle. The splenic flexure is totally released, and the non-irradiated descending colon is mobilized for coloanal anastomosis

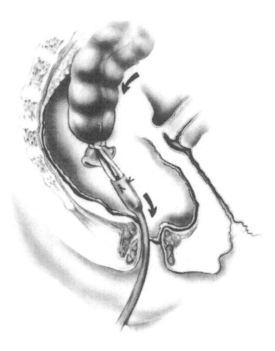

Fig. 6. With the aid of the red rubber catheter, the non-irradiated descending colon is guided through the anal canal, ensuring proper orientation

antibiotic-soaked sponge, and the pelvis is filled with antibiotic solution. The inferior mesenteric artery and vein are isolated, and the vein is ligated and interrupted prior to ligating the artery close to its origin. The inferior mesenteric vein will be interrupted again at the level of the duodenojejunal junction as the depth of the mesentery is stepped to provide adequate mobilization and length of colon. The ascending branch of the left colic artery and the left branch of the middle colic artery are customarily interrupted. This is performed deep in the mesentery to avoid disturbing the marginal artery (Fig. 5).

The site for transection of the descending colon proximal to the previously placed black silk suture is determined and the mesentery incised to that point. Diverticula, which may have been noted on the barium enema study, should be avoided. The length of bowel necessary to reach the anal canal without tension is determined by a rule of thumb requiring the bowel to lie a comfortable five-fingers breadth distal to the symphysis pubis. A stout cloth tape is tied securely 2 cm proximal to a bowel clamp marking the point of transection. The knot on the tape is generally placed in the left posterior position for subsequent orientation after transection. The bowel is transected and the specimen removed from the fold. The end of the bowel is carefully cleansed, covered with a washed glove, and the tape brought through a slit in one of the fingers. The red rubber catheter is retrieved from the pelvis, and

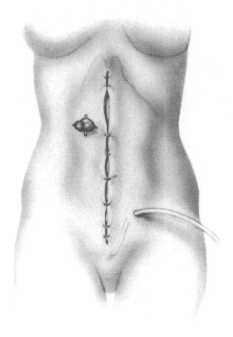

Fig. 7. A temporary diverting transverse loop colostomy is created, suction drainage of the pelvis is established, and the abdominal incision is closed in standard fashion

the tape is sutured into its open end. Following this, the glove finger is brought over the catheter and tied. An assistant moves to the perineal field and places gentle traction on the catheter while the operating surgeon assists by pressing and guiding the bowel into the pelvic floor (Fig. 6). The descending colon is passed, rather than pulled, into the pelvis. When the bowel exits the anal canal, it is properly oriented by the knot placement, and the catheter is fixed with a clamp. Following the exchange of gowns, gloves, and instruments, the abdomen is redraped and lavaged. A proximal loop transverse colostomy is created and a suction catheter inserted to drain the pelvis, following which the abdomen is closed and the supported colostomy opened and matured (Fig. 7). By preference, unless there are high-density diverticula in the transverse colon, a diverting loop ileostomy is avoided inasmuch as the small bowel may have been exposed to irradiation.

Upon securing the abdominal dressings, the exaggerated lithotomy position is reassumed. The rubber glove covering the bowel is carefully teased out of the anal canal and pelvis, and the anterior wall of exteriorized bowel is opened transversely from the right to the left lateral positions. The anastomosis is conducted by slight eversion of the anal canal and insertion of a zero-gauge absorbable suture placed first in the anterior midline and held (Fig. 8). Stout purchases of both the colon and the anal canal wall are consid-

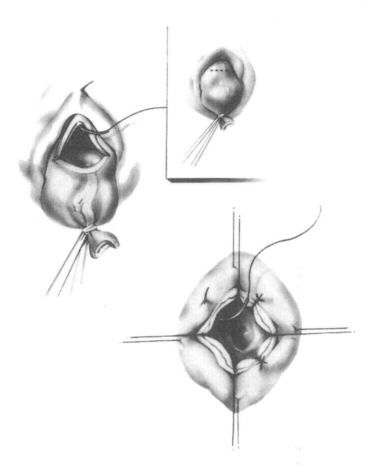

Fig. 8. The exaggerated lithotomy position is re-established and a cuffless, handsewn anastomosis is created with care taken to obtain full thickness of the bowel and a stout purchase of the anal canal wall

ered important. Similar cardinal sutures are placed in the right and left lateral positions and held as well. The transection of the bowel is then completed posteriorly, and the last cardinal suture is placed in the posterior midline and held. It is important to avoid inserting a finger or instrument through the anal canal into the pelvis during this period for fear of contamination. Four intervening sutures are placed in the same manner and tied sequentially. The cardinal sutures are tied to complete the anastomosis. The anastomosis may be checked and additional sutures inserted if required – an uncommon necessity.

Perioperative Management

Systemic antibiotics are given for no less than 14 days postoperatively because it is our belief that the radiated field is more susceptible to anaerobic infection. The suction catheters are usually removed before the 3rd or 4th day, and it is not uncommon for a small issue of serous fluid to exit through the anal canal between the 4th and 7th day. Irrigation with tap water through the distal stoma begins in the 3rd postoperative week. Digital examination is not performed until the 5th postoperative week, but not delayed beyond the 6th week if stenosis is to be avoided. A water-soluble contrast study performed through the distal stoma is accomplished in the 5th week coincidental to digital rectal examination. Careful narrow-lumen rigid sigmoidoscopy is also performed, allowing inspection for any evidence of purulence, which may be the only hint of a small anastomotic defect. Closure of the stoma is never performed before the 8th postoperative week and only after direct inspection and radiographic studies indicate satisfactory healing.

It is mandatory that every digital and rigid sigmoidoscopic examination be conducted with great care. A thoughtlessly rough digital or endoscopic examination may disrupt the anastomosis, an event we have seen occur as much as 18 months postoperatively. Forewarning patients that, immediately after colostomy closure, diarrhea accompanied by temporary incontinence is commonplace may help avoid emotional trauma. Accommodation to the loss of reservoir rectal function and to the shortened and irradiated bowel requires dietary and antidiarrheal measures, as well as patience. Maintaining a lactose-free diet is critical.

Evaluation of the patient is carried out at 3-month intervals. Digital examination with documentation of extrarectal configuration is desirable to better ensure accurate interpretation of any future findings when recurrence is in question. Routine visits are at 3-month intervals for 2 years, then at 4-month intervals until the 5th year, after which 6-month intervals are followed. Carcinoembryonic antigen levels are determined at each visit. Chest roentgenography, CT, and MRI of the abdomen and pelvis are performed selectively, as is endorectal and endovaginal sonography. Intramural and extrarectal abnormal masses are subjected to endoscopic or CT-guided needle biopsy. Flexible sigmoidoscopy can be carried out at 6-month intervals, and colonoscopy at prescribed surveillance intervals. Anal competence is evaluated according to Park's criteria (1975), which define difficulty in controlling flatus or acute attacks of diarrhea as being within the range of acceptable function.

Results

Of the first 82 patients treated by the TATA procedure, 65 had rectal cancers at or below the 3-cm level. Sixty-six percent were men, and the ages ranged from 29 to 83 years, with a median age of 59. Level in the rectum is shown

Table 1. Level of cancers in the rectum ($n=65$)

Level (cm)	Number	%
3.0–2.1	24	37
2.0–1.1	25	38
1.0–0.5	16	25

Table 2. Post-irradiation pathological stage and local recurrence rates ($n=65$)

Stage	Local recurrence No./total	%
$\leq T_2$	0/35	0
$\leq T_2 \pm N$	0/44	0
$\geq T_3 \pm N$	6/21	29
All	6/65	9

in Table 1. Post-irradiation pathological stage and local recurrence rates are shown in Table 2.

Twenty of 65 (31%) of the cancers were fixed at the time of initial examination but became mobile following irradiation. The exclusion of cancers that remain fixed after radiation meant that this select group of patients has a higher percentage of favorable tumors (35/65, 54%) than the series as a whole (78/203, 38%).

Significant perioperative radiation-related morbidity was nonexistent. Radiation therapy was interrupted briefly in less than 5% of patients because of diarrhea. One patient developed a wound infection that responded to drainage and antibiotics; three significant pelvic abscesses occurred, all responding to percutaneous drainage. One major anastomotic disruption occurred and has never been reconstituted. There was one radiographically demonstrated leak that healed spontaneously, in which diverticula were presumed to be the source. Mild anastomotic mucosal adhesions were frequent and easily managed by digital dilatation. One individual experienced incontinence attributed to a previously unrecognized obstetrically induced disruption that was repaired with short-lived benefit. There was one perioperative death from a pulmonary embolus 55 days after surgery, constituting the only surgical mortality in the entire program.

Age was found to be a factor in the quality of continence. Function is determined by clinical assessment and was satisfactory in all but 5% of patients. There was 100% follow-up in our patients. Six of the 65 (9%) of patients developed local recurrence. The rate of recurrence was less than in the entire series, 22/203 (11%). There were no local recurrences among those with post-irradiation favorable-stage (T2 or less) cancers, even surprisingly, if nodes were involved (Table 2). Kaplan-Meier 5-year actuarial survival for the group is 85%.

Conclusion

The results of this prospective program of high-dose preoperative radiation therapy and the transanal abdominal transanal radical proctosigmoidectomy with direct coloanal anastomosis (TATA) for select cancers of the distal 3 cm of the rectum establishes the feasibility of radical sphincter preservation surgery with coloanal anastomosis after irradiation for cancers at the very lowest level of the rectum. The improved survival and reduced local recurrence rate accomplished with minimal morbidity and mortality attest to the quality of life benefits of a selective multimodality approach to the patient with a post-irradiation nonfixed distal rectal cancer.

It is our conviction that the salutary results observed in this study accrue both from the features related to the technique of the TATA and the effect of the preoperative external irradiation upon the primary cancer and the microlymphatics.

References

Ahmad N, Marks G, Mohiuddin M (1993) High-dose preoperative radiation for cancer of the rectum: impact of radiation dose on patterns of failure and survival. Int J Radiat Oncol Biol Phys 27:773–778

Marks G (1973) Rectal reconstruction by a combined adominotranssacral approach: report of three cases. Dis Colon Rectum 16:378–382

Marks G (1976) Combined abdominotranssacral reconstruction of the radiation injured rectum. Am J Surg 131:54–59

Marks G, Mohiuddin M, Borenstein B (1985) Preoperative radiation therapy and sphincter preservation by the combined abdominotranssacral technique for selected rectal cancers. Dis Colon Rectum 28:565–571

Marks G, Mohiuddin M, Masoni L, Montori A (1992) High-dose preoperative radiation therapy as the key to extending sphincter-preservation surgery for cancer of the distal rectum. Surg Oncol Clin North Am 1:71–86

Mendenhall WM, Million RR, Bland KI et al. (1985) Preoperative radiation therapy for clinically resectable adenocarcinoma of the rectum. Ann Surg 202:215–221

Parks AG (1975) Anorectal incontinence. Proc R Soc Med 68:681–690

Radiochemotherapy and Hyperthermia in the Treatment of Rectal Cancer*

P. Wust[1], B. Rau[2], J. Gellermann[1], W. Pegios[1], J. Löffel[3], H. Riess[3], R. Felix[1], and P. M. Schlag[2]

[1] Department of Radiation Oncology, Charité Medical School – Campus-Virchow-Klinikum, Humboldt University, 13344 Berlin, Germany
[2] Department of Surgery, Charité Medical School – Campus Berlin-Buch, Humboldt University, 13122 Berlin, Germany
[3] Department of Medical Oncology, Charité Medical School – Campus Virchow-Klinikum, Humboldt University, 13344 Berlin, Germany

Abstract

We evaluated the use of regional hyperthermia with radio-chemotherapy in a phase I/II study on locally advanced rectal carcinomas. Thirty-four patients with primary advanced (stage T3/T4) rectal carcinomas (24 patients) or recurring rectal carcinomas (6 patients) were treated using preoperative radio-chemo-thermotherapy. Initial tumour staging was carried out clinically (degree of fixation) and using endorectal ultrasonography and CT. Radiotherapy was carried out with the patient prone (on a belly board) at 5 × 1.8 Gy per week up to 45 Gy at the reference point. 5-Fluorouracil (300–500 mg/m^2) was administered with low-dose leucovorin (50 mg) on days 1–5 and 22–26. Patients were treated with regional hyperthermia each week prior to radiotherapy, using the Sigma-60 ring of the BSD-2000 system. Temperature/position curves and temperature/time curves were recorded via endocavitary catheters (tumour contact, bladder, vagina). Following endosonographic and clinical restaging, the operation was carried out 4–6 weeks after the end of preoperative therapy. In cases where tumours were unresectable, a boost of up to 60 Gy was given. Twenty-three of the 34 patients (68%) proved to be curatively resectable. Of these patients, 70% were downstaged endosonographically during preoperative therapy. The actuarial survival rates among these patients were 85% (primary rectal cancer) and 60% (recurrences) at 30 months. All in all, the preoperative multimodal therapy was well tolerated, and premature termination was necessary in only two cases. The quality of temperature distribution (T_{90}, cum min T_{90} > 40.5°C) depends on the power level and relative power density. The response (particularly downstaging) correlates significantly with the quality parameters of the temperature distributions. This regimen proved practical and effective, with encouraging downstaging rates and local control rates.

---

* This work is supported by the Deutsche Forschungsgemeinschaft, Sonderforschungsbereich 273, and Berliner Sparkassenstiftung Medizin.

Introduction

In cases of locally advanced or recurrent rectal cancer further optimization and intensification of local therapy is required even though preoperative high-dose radiotherapy (with or without chemotherapy) and subsequent curative surgery generally achieves quite favourable results. In a high-risk group of patients with fixed and/or distally located tumours or tumour recurrence, local control is still unsatisfactory, with local failure rates of 20%–50% even after combined curative surgery and radio- and chemotherapy (Ahmad et al. 1993; Minsky et al. 1993). The prognosis for locally advanced, tumours which remain unresectable after preoperative multimodal therapy is especially depressing (Emami et al. 1982).

Hyperthermia is a new supplemental modality in cancer therapy involving raising the temperature in tumours up to 40 °C and higher. Temperatures of 42–43 °C are desired.

Regional hyperthermia may improve the local effectiveness of radio- and chemotherapy. Significant improvement in local control has already been demonstrated in several European phase III studies when hyperthermia is added to radiotherapy in the treatment of malignant regional metastases of melanomas (Overgaard et al. 1995), recurrent breast cancer (Vernon et al. 1994), and pelvic tumors (van der Zee et al. 1995).

The old Greek physicians such as Hippocrates knew that heat has a curative effect on diseases. Hippocrates reported: What drugs cannot cure, can be cured by surgery; what surgery cannot cure, can be cured by hyperthermia; what hyperthermia cannot cure, is incurable.

Today, basic science gives a precise rationale for the use of heat in cancer therapy (Streffer 1995). Numerous potential applications have been derived from preclinical experiments documenting such phenomena as synergism with radiotherapy (Konings 1995) and chemotherapy (Dahl 1995), direct cytotoxic effects modulated by factors in the physiological milieu and, finally, induction of protein synthesis or activation which can induce or modulate regulation, e.g. immunoregulatory mechanisms (stimulation, depression).

Heat has a cytocidal effect which is demonstrated in Fig. 1. Survival curves for heat are similar in shape to those for radiation. The cell-kill effect depends on temperature and time. A thermal dose can be derived which is a kind of temperature-time product. Figure 1a illustrates an important phenomenon: that thermo-tolerance occurs if the cells are heated to lower temperatures for some time. Dose-response relationships vary from cell to cell. For example, Fig. 1b gives data for cell line SW 620, which is much more sensitive to high temperatures than cell line WiDr (Fig. 1a).

A particularly important point is that heat potentiates radiotherapy and some chemotherapeutic agents as well. These drugs are cisplatin, ifosfamide, doxorubicin, ACNU, BCNU, etoposide, mitoxantrone, bleomycin and the interferons, among others. For example, a potentiation of effectiveness by a factor of 10^5 can be seen for cisplatin, if the temperature rises from 37 °C to 43 °C.

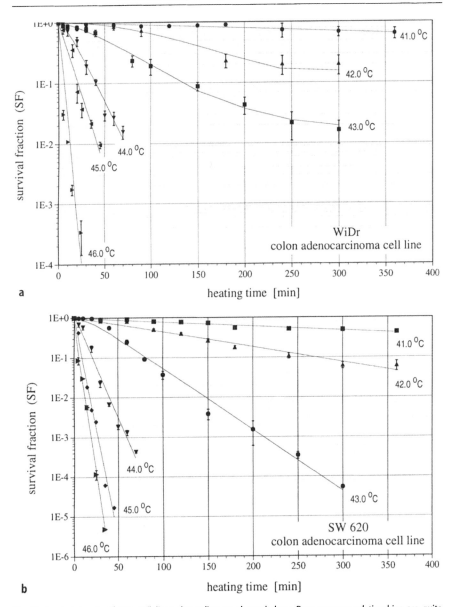

Fig. 1. Survival curves of two cell lines depending on thermal dose. Dose-response-relationships are quite different between cell lines (Jordan et al. 1996)

To summarize the preconditions for applying heat in patients in the clinical setting and what we know from preclinical research, we have looked for the following phenomena: cytotoxicity, sensitization or potentiation and regulation mechanisms, e.g. in the immune system. Our laboratory tools are in vivo studies on cell cultures, in vitro studies on experimental tumours and

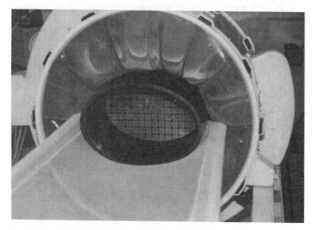

Fig. 2. Sigma-60 phased-array applicator of the BSD-2000 system. An elliptical phantom with a visualizing lamp matrix is positioned in the ring. The water bolus is required to couple the power into the tissue of the patient

the sophisticated tools of molecular biology, particularly analyses of proteins and RNA.

Encouraging preclinical data formed the rationale for using hyperthermia in clinical practice. Local hyperthermia is a heating technique for superficial tumours. Obviously, heating superficial tumours is relatively easy compared to heating deep-seated tumours.

If hyperthermia is employed to treat tumours in patients, a method of temperature measurement is required. For the purpose of thermometry catheters are implanted in tumours under CT guidance. Small thermistors are inserted in these catheters during heat treatment. These sensors can be moved stepwise along the catheter on demand at certain intervals during therapy.

The temperature measurements are used to define thermal variables (Dewhirst 1995). T_{min} is a time average minimum temperature in the tumour. T_x is the so-called index temperature which is reached or exceeded in x% of the temperature measurement points. Temperature/position curves are evaluated with respect to the index temperatures. One can also look for the time we reach a certain T_{90} in a tumour (cumulative minutes), or even calculate an equivalent time with respect to a reference temperature (usually 43 °C). As a rule of thumb one can say: for every 1 °C increase in temperature, the time can be halved for an equivalent biological effect on the tumour.

These thermal variables have been correlated successfully with clinical outcome, especially response or local control. The existence of a correlation between heat treatment and therapeutic outcome is confirmation of the effectiveness of clinical hyperthermia. Among other groups in our clinic, a correlation of this kind between achieved index temperatures and response has been determined for advanced neck node metastases of head and neck carcinomas (Wust et al. 1996a) and rectal carcinomas (see below) as well.

Hyperthermia of deep-seated tumours, e.g. in the pelvic region, is considerably more difficult. The most advanced and popular system for hyperthermia of deep-seated tumours is shown in Fig. 2, with an elliptical phantom for visualization of power distributions. An annular phased array applicator, the Sigma-60 applicator, is used to generate a power deposition pattern in the body. Antennae surround the patient. Electromagnetic waves in the radiofrequency range – in this case 90 MHz – are radiated by these antennae and coupled by a water bolus to the target volume.

An important tool to understanding complex hyperthermia systems like the annular phased array applicator is the phantom in Fig. 2. (Wust et al. 1996b). This phantom with a fat-equivalent wall is positioned in the ring applicator like a patient. In the central plane an array of lamps is arranged emitting light in correlation with the electrical field strength.

Figure 3 illustrates a typical behaviour of a deep-seated tumour as seen on CT scan. It shows a locally advanced rectal cancer before and after a multimodal treatment regimen. To monitor the heat treatment a thermometry catheter was endoluminally inserted into this tumour. Temperatures were measured in contact with the tumour. The rectal carcinoma was dorsally located, so the maximum power was shifted to the bottom of the phantom. A phase delay on the bottom channel entails a shift of the pattern in the direction of this delay. Unfortunately, in the three-dimensional heterogeneous tissue of a real patient these promising conditions cannot be obtained.

Hyperthermia has been used clinically as an adjunct to radiotherapy for about 10–15 years. In the beginning, phase II studies strongly suggested that hyperthermia might be effective in improving local control. Matched pair analyses mean that comparable tumour lesions in the same patient are stratified to treatment with radiotherapy alone or combined radio- and thermotherapy. In all these studies the number of complete remissions more than doubles when hyperthermia is added (Overgaard et al. 1989). Comparison of the combined therapy with historical controls also indicated a strong superiority of the combination therapy.

Recently, a couple of phase III studies were completed which confirm the biological effectiveness of hyperthermia (Valdagni et al. 1993; Vernon et al. 1994; van der Zee et al. 1995). However, here a problem with hyperthermia was also found. The first randomized hyperthermia study on superficial tumours in the United States (Radiotherapeutic Oncology Group Study no. 81-04), failed. Retrospective analysis revealed that the quality of the hyperthermia was weak and most of the heat treatments were technically inadequate (Perez et al. 1989). Only for a sub-group of smaller tumours (less than 3 cm) was an advantage of combined treatment proven in this study. The same happened with the third study of the European Society of Hyperthermic Oncology in advanced breast cancer, where techniques were also inadequate. However, three other studies showed clearly improved local control in the combined treatment group (for neck node metastases, melanoma metastases and recurrent breast cancer). Two other studies dealt with deep-seated tumours. One of the Netherland's groups, the Rotterdam Group, also demonstrated the

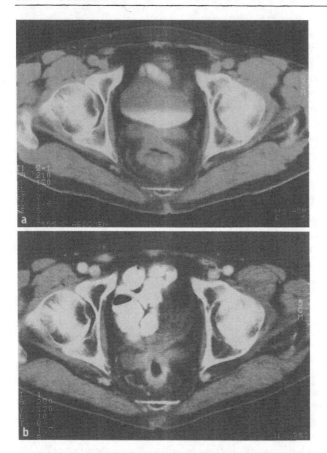

Fig. 3a, b. CT scans before and after multimodal therapy according the schema shown in Fig. 4. A locally advanced rectal cancer stage uT4 (seminal vesicle, dorsal bladder wall) undergoes considerable volume reduction

effectiveness of regional hyperthermia using the Sigma applicator, the one that we use in our study (van der Zee et al. 1995).

Thus, both preclinical and clinical studies offer a strong rationale for the use of hyperthermia in cancer therapy (Wust et al. 1995).

We started clinical research into hyperthermia in 1989. Most of the tumours treated in the first period in our department were very extensive and recurrent tumours. Up to 1995, 300 patients had been treated in about 1500 heat sessions, most of them with rectal carcinomas, cervical carcinomas, soft tissue sarcomas and lymph node metastases from head and neck carcinomas. Based upon this clinical experience, three randomized studies on deep-seated tumours have now been started in Germany. One study deals with rectal cancer and is the subject of the rest of this article.

Design and Results of a Phase I/II Study

In the period from April 1993 to September 1995, 30 patients (25 male, 5 female) with primary advanced stage T3/T4 rectal carcinomas (24 patients) or recurring rectal carcinomas (6 patients) were treated with preoperative radio-chemo-thermotherapy. Median age was 59 years (range 31–75 years). Patient characteristics are shown in Table 1. Regional hyperthermia (once a week) was included in a standard preoperative scheme of radio-chemotherapy (Fig. 4).

Radiotherapy was performed with the patient prone on a belly-board using a three-field technique with additional individual blockings, aiming at 45 Gy in the reference point. Chemotherapy was administered on days 1–5 and 22–26, starting with leucovorin 50 mg as a short infusion, followed by 5-FU 300 mg/m^2 as a bolus.

Regional hyperthermia was induced with the radiofrequency annular phased array system BSD-2000 using the ring applicator Sigma 60 (BSD Medical Corp., Salt Lake City, Utah). We usually selected a standard set-up (90 MHz, 20°–40° phase delay in the dorsal pair of antennae). A corresponding power distribution obtained by a three-dimensional calculation (Nadobny et al. 1996, Wust et al. 1993, 1996) is shown in Fig. 5. Thermometry was car-

Table 1. Patient characteristics in the phase II study

	Tumour stage[a]		Recurrence after	
	uT3 n = 12	uT4 n = 12	Anterior resection n = 4	Abdomino-perineal resection n = 2
Mason stage				
2 (tethered)	1	–	–	–
3 (fixed)	4	2	2	–
4 (advanced fixation)	5	7	–	–
Data not available	2	3	2	2
Tumour level (from anal verge)				
0–5 cm	6	5	–	–
5–10 cm	3	4	1	–
10–16 cm	3	3	2	–
Data not available	–	–	1	2
Resectability (estimated)				
Potentially resectable	5	1	–	–
Unresectable	7	11	4	2
Lymph nodes				
N–	4	6	4	2
N+	8	6	–	–

[a] As determined by endorectal ultrasonography.

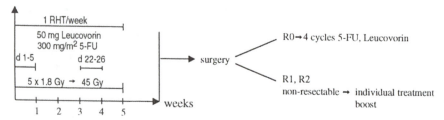

Fig. 4. Schema of the neoadjuvant therapy study (radio-chemo-thermotherapy) with adjuvant chemotherapy after curative surgery. RHT, Regional hyperthermia

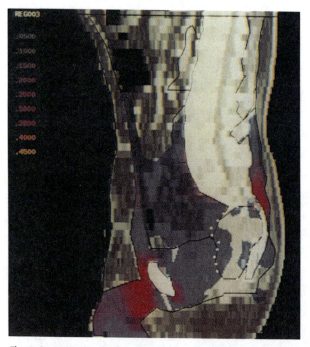

Fig. 5. Power distribution for a standard setup in regional hyperthermia of rectal cancer. Hot spots at pubic symphysis and dorsal sacral bone in a 3D calculation (power distribution in sagittal plane)

ried out via endoluminally inserted catheters in contact with the tumour or (after rectum extirpation) in intratumorally implanted catheters with Bowman thermistors (see Fig. 3). Temperature scans along catheters in tumour contact are analysed in relation to index temperature T_x, T_{max} and cum min $T_{90} \geq 40.5\,°C$ (cumulative time during which T_{90} remained above $40.5\,°C$ in a heat treatment, see above).

Acute toxicity of regional hyperthermia is mainly caused by E field elevations at electrical boundaries (fat/muscle, bone/muscle interfaces), so-called hot spot phenomena (see Fig. 5), resulting in local discomfort or pain sensations occasionally persisting hours to days after heat treatment. Systemic side effects proved to be minor. Of course, the heat treatment is generally stressful and uncomfortable (bolus pressure), requiring a good level of patient motivation.

In the course of our long clinical experience a toxicity score for regional hyperthermia has been developed following established toxicity scores (WHO score, Lent Soma tables) (Table 2). The acute toxicity of the preoperative regimen (related to radiotherapy or chemotherapy) was acceptable. Grade III toxicity occurred in less than 20% of patients in skin and intestine, and were reduced by slightly decreasing the chemotherapy dosage and developing a special cooling device for the rima ani (where the skin reaction is most typically expressed).

Grade III toxicity specific for the heat treatment was defined by refusal of further heat treatment after 1-2 sessions and occurred in about 10% of cases.

Overall 14/18 (78%) of unresectable primary rectal carcinomas and 2/6 (33%) of recurrent rectal carcinomas became curatively resectable. Table 3 gives further information about the surgical procedures performed. Note the difference between the endorectal sonographic "u" classification and the assessment of resectability by the surgeon (mainly according to the degree of fixation, see Table 1).

Perioperative complications were moderate and comparable to those occurring after surgery alone (Table 4). Only disturbances of perineal wound healing were increased by preoperative irradiation.

Two long-term complications causing death occurred in the unresectable rectal cancer group (one rectum perforation, one intestinal-cutaneous fistula, both resulting in septic failure), where interference between tumour-related effects (infiltration, destruction) and treatment-related effects (after 60 Gy irradiation) may have occurred.

Response to the combined treatment was evaluated according to WHO criteria in relation to tumour volume as assessed by CT, MRI or clinical examination: complete remission (CR), partial remission (PR), no change (NC) or

Table 2. Toxicity score for regional radiofrequency hyperthermia[a]

Grade 0:	General discomfort (bolus pressure, systemic stress); no limitation of heat treatment
Grade I:	Local discomfort (hot spot phenomena, positioning problems or systemic stress) which requires rearrangement of treatment set-up; heat treatment can be accomplished with some restrictions in total power and power distribution
Grade II:	More severe local discomfort or systemic stress which persists after end of heat treatment or evidently limits effectiveness
Grade III:	Any kind of toxicity that causes the patient to refuse further heat treatments (hot spots, musculo-skeletal syndrome, claustrophobia, etc.)
Grade IV:	Burns, tissue damage, systemic collapse or any other complications related to the heat treatment

[a] Sigma-60 phased array applicator, BSD-2000 system

Table 3. Surgical procedures in relation to the different tumour stages

uT3 12/30 (40%)	12/12 curative resections
	< 6 cm: 6/12 4 APR
	2 continence preservation
	> 6 cm: 6/12 6 continence preservation
Result: 7/7 unresectable tumours become resectable	
uT4 12/30 (40%)	8/12 curative resections
	< 6 cm: 3/8 2 APR
	1 continence preservation
	> 6 cm: 5/8 5 continence preservation
	4/12 unresectable: 3 explorative laparotomy
	1 clinical criteria
Result: 7/11 unresectable tumours become resectable	
Recurrent 6/30 (20%)	1/6 anterior resection
	1/6 APR
	1/6 surgery refused
	3/6 unresectable: 2 explorative laparotomy
	1 clinical criteria
Result: 2/6 unresectable tumours become resectable	

APR, Abdomino-perineal resection

Table 4. Perioperative and postoperative (long-term) complications

Perioperative complications	
(22 curative resections, 5 explorative laparatomies)	
Pneumonia	2
Cardial dysrhythmia	1
Urinary retention	1
Anastomotic leakage	2
Abdominal wound infection	1
Perineal wound infection	3
Perineal abscess	3
Stoma revision	1
Long-term complications/toxicity	
Intestinal obstruction	1
Rectum perforation (after 60 Gy)	1
Intestinal cutaneous fistula (after 60 Gy)	1
Sexual dysfunction in male (erectility, ejaculation)	4
Sexual dysfunction in female (dyspareunia)	1

Table 5. Overall response after radio-chemo-thermotherapy in the phase II study in 30 patients (WHO classification)

Tumour stage	No.	%	
uT3 (n=12)			
CR	1	8	
PR	6	50	
NC	5	42	
uT4 (n=12)			
CR	1	8	CR 13%
PR	6	50	PR 50%
NC	3	25	NC 27%
PD	2	17	PD 10%
Recurrence (n=6)			
CR	2	33	
PR	3	50	
PD	1	17	
Response: 63%			

progressive disease (PD). Furthermore, in the patient group undergoing curative tumour resection PR is also recorded if a downstaging from the initial uT classification to the histopathological pT classification is documented (especially CR in the case of pT0).

The response rate of 63% in the whole group is encouraging. The CR rate was 4/30 (i.e. 13%). Specifically, in the group with resected tumours a histopathologically proven downstaging of 59% emerged. Response is summarized in Table 5 and Fig. 6.

Resectability and response in our phase II study are compared with two other recently published phase II studies by Chan et al. (1993) and Chen et al. (1994) in Table 6. The results of our study (comparing the distribution of pT stages in the resected specimens) appear quite favourable, especially if initial clinical stage (recurrent or fixed in Chan et al. 1993) and radiation dose (56 Gy in Chen et al. 1994) are considered.

In a slightly larger group of 34 patients where response was evaluable (four of them had to be excluded from the phase II study) thermal parameters were determined and correlated with response. A statistical description of thermal parameters in 34 patients (measured in contact with the tumour) is given in Table 7. A significant correlation of the averaged T_{90} and cum min $T_{90} \geq 40.5\,°C$ with response can be shown. This important result indicates that endoluminal temperature measurements (in tumour contact) are suitable for estimating the effectiveness of heat treatment. In consequence, invasive thermometry, which is unpleasant to the patient and adds toxicity, could be avoidable. This conclusion can be generalized to cervical cancer, bladder cancer, prostate cancer and anal cancer.

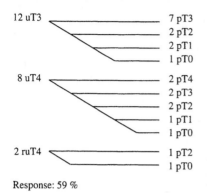

Response: 59 %

Fig. 6. Histopathological response after radio-chemo-thermotherapy in 22 patients with curative resection

Table 6. Comparison of different phase II studies of treatment for rectal cancer with preoperative treatment schemes

	Chan et al. (1993) ($n=46$) %	Chen et al. (1994) ($n=31$) %	Present study ($n=30$) %
Curative resection	89	100	73
Fixed tumour	35	100	97
Tethered tumour	65	0	3
Recurrent tumour	0	0	20
Stage after curative resection:			
pT0	5	10	14
pT1	5	0	14
pT2	49	32	23
pT3	34	42	40
pT4	7	16	9
Preop. radiation dose	40 Gy	56 Gy	40–45 Gy
5-Fluorouracil dose	20 mg/m^2 +mitomycin C	200-300 mg/m^2 continuously	300-500 mg/m^2 +50 mg leucovorin

Local control after preoperative combined therapy and curative resection in 22 patients was excellent (100% in a median observation time of 18 months), with only one local progression outside the treatment volume (para-aortic). Local control in 8 patients with unresectable tumours (after preoperative therapy) was less good (<40% in 10–27 months), and local failure is the predominant cause of death in this patient group. Therefore, a more effective local therapy is still needed for these patients with unresectable tumours.

Overall survival is 85% for primary rectal cancer (24 patients) and 60% for recurrent rectal cancer in a median observation period of 16 months (Fig. 7). Disease-free survival is slightly above 60% for primary rectal cancer and 40% for recurrences.

Table 7. Mean values of thermal and power-related parameters

T_{90}	40.4 (38.9–41.4) °C
T_{max}	41.4 (40.4–42.3) °C
Cum min $T_{90} \geq 40.5$ °C (per heat treatment)	27 (0–80) min
Cum min $T_{90} \geq 40.5$ °C (per patient)	123 (0–330) min
Total power	660 (350–1000) W
Specific absorption rate	32.3 (12.0–79.5) mW/g

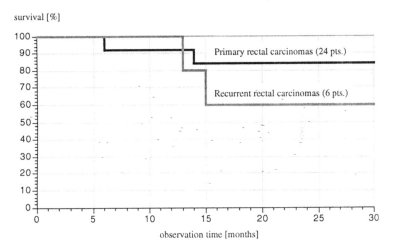

Fig. 7. Survival plot (Kaplan-Meier) stratified according to primary and recurrent rectal cancers

Discussion

Preoperative combined radio- and chemotherapy has been tested in locally advanced rectal carcinomas (clinically fixed, ≥T3) in phase II studies (Chan et al. 1993; Chen et al. 1994), and is currently the subject of phase III studies (e.g. an EORTC study), However, there are risk groups in whom local control is still unsatisfactory, despite multimodal therapy. For example, the local recurrence rate for fixed tumours (Mason III) is 20% in spite of preoperative radiotherapy and curative surgery. When fixation is advanced (Mason IV), this rises to 50% (Mohiuddin et al. 1993). Another risk factor is distal tumour location, with local recurrence rates of 20%–30%. In cases where the tumour remains unresectable the prognosis is extremely bad, and most patients die within 2–3 years from local progression (Dosoretz et al. 1983). The rate of complete remission following high-dose preoperative radiotherapy or radio-chemotherapy is only 0–20% – still unsatisfactorily low. To improve local control at least in these risk groups, preoperative therapy has to be intensified. This has been done using, for example, intraoperative radiotherapy (Gunderson et al. 1992).

In the phase II study presented here, regional radiowave hyperthermia was used in addition to preoperative radio-chemotherapy. In cases of advanced inoperable pelvic tumours (cervical, bladder, rectal carcinoma), the same hyperthermia system has already made significant improvements to the complete remission rate (37% after radiotherapy alone, 58% after combined radio- and chemotherapy) (van der Zee et al. 1995). Other studies of hyperthermia in rectal carcinoma (Mori et al. 1989; Berdov and Menteshashvili 1990; You et al. 1993) were performed using endocavitary methods, and are therefore difficult to compare; but hyperthermia was still shown to improve the effects of radiotherapy.

The high downstaging rate of 70% achieved on curatively operated patients in this study cannot be compared with the published results of other groups where these groups did not carry out pretreatment staging by endorectal ultrasonography. Nevertheless, Table 6 groups patients by histopathological stages in this study together with two other phase II studies of preoperative radiochemotherapy in patient series taken to be comparable. Our results appear very positive, especially when one considers the large number of recurrent and fixed tumours in our own series in relation to the low pT stages in the resected specimens. Local control is still 100% in the curatively operated patients after an observation period of up to 30 months, whereas in the series of Chan et al. (1993), the actuarial local recurrence rate after 30 months in the group of patients with initially fixed rectal carcinomas was 40%. At 14%, the number of complete remissions lies in the upper region of the best that can be expected with preoperative radiochemotherapy. Naturally, this is not proof of the effectiveness of hyperthermia. For that we need a phase III study comparing radiochemotherapy with radiochemothermotherapy; such a study has already begun.

By abandoning invasive intratumoral temperature measurement, regional hyperthermia has been made much more gentle than before, and it has become better accepted by both patients and the medical profession. We have demonstrated (Table 7) that endoluminal temperature measurement with tumour contact allows the effectiveness of regional hyperthermia to be assessed. As in the study by Issels et al. 1990 (see Leopold et al. 1993; Wust et al. 1996a), quality parameters of temperature measurement points in tumour contact (T_{90}, cum min $T_{90} \geq 40.5\,°C$) correlated with the downstaging rate in curatively operated patients, as well as with local control of unresectable rectal carcinomas. This demonstrates that opting against intratumoral (invasive) temperature measurements is justified. Similar arguments can be used against invasive temperature measurement in cervical, bladder and prostate carcinomas.

High relative specific absorption rate (SAR) values proved predictive of good T_{90} and cum min $T_{90} \geq 40.5\,°C$ (Wust et al. 1996a). It is therefore a good idea to attempt to increase the SAR values in the tumour region as much as possible by suitably manipulating the SAR distribution. The numerous parameters that influence this distribution include the phase and amplitude of the various channels, geometric factors (patient position, tilt, position of central plane), as well as factors linked with shielding and coupling measures. The most effective strategy for increasing the SAR in the tumour region is reducing the hot spots, as this allows the total power to be increased. The main ways of reducing hot spots are shielding, and perhaps greatly reducing the amplitude of the nearest channel. Systematic analysis of the control of SAR distributions using antenna systems is the subject of basic methodical research, particularly in modern planning systems (Seebass et al. 1995; Wust et al. 1996b).

Interestingly, total power is affected by something we did not expect: low total powers correlate with better temperature distributions. Perfusion and thermoregulation in the tumour obviously play an important role here. If there is little or no thermoregulation, temperatures of 41 °C and more are achieved at low total power levels, thus allowing good temperature distributions with low total power. Conversely, if thermoregulation is sufficient, even increasing the power sometimes fails to produce satisfactory temperature distribution. This matches our clinical experience that hyperthermia is more difficult in young, active patients who have large reserves for increasing their cardiac output. Surprisingly, regional hyperthermia has often proven simple and comfortable for older patients, as therapeutic temperatures can be reached at low power levels. It is conceivable that controlling cardiac output, which would include influencing psychological factors, is just as important to regional hyperthermia as optimising the power distribution.

The pre-clinical rationale for hyperthermia has been known for a long time. As well as its cytotoxic and sensitising effects, other reasons for its effectiveness have been under discussion recently. In particular, hyperthermia can lead to reoxygenation (possibly by raising perfusion), which improves the effects of radiotherapy (Oleson 1995). This might explain why benefits have been obtained at low temperatures (T_{90} approximately 40–40.5 °C), even though these temperatures are unlikely to damage cells under in vivo conditions, i.e. when perfused (Hentschel et al. 1997).

In this phase II study, a multi-modal therapy regime with acceptable toxicity was found for the advanced and recurrent rectal carcinomas. Hyperthermia was used as part of the regime and, once the rima ani cooling system had been introduced, did not increase the side effects of radiotherapy and chemotherapy. The downstaging rates and survival curves are so encouraging (including when compared with data in the literature) that continued evaluation of regional hyperthermia in a phase III study is justified. We also hope that regional hyperthermia will continue to undergo technical development, beginning with optimisation of planning systems and endocavitary support for hyperthermia by a hot water flow-through system (hot source principle) or endocavitary antennae. Influencing the patients systemically, e.g. using thermal insulation, may also improve hyperthermia clinically.

Conclusions

Combined preoperative treatment with radio- and chemotherapy and hyperthermia carries acceptable acute toxicity (grade III < 20%). Perioperative complications are moderate and not increased by hyperthermia. Resectability (about 80% of primary rectal cancers initially assessed as unresectable), response rate (about 60%) and local control (100% for curatively resected tumours, 40% for unresectable tumours in a median observation period of 16 months) are encouraging. Thermal parameters T_{90}, cum min $T_{90} > 40.5\,°C$ derived from endoluminally measured temperature scans correlate with response. The technology for regional hyperthermia (BSD-2000) is suitable for heating deep-seated pelvic tumours effectively, but still needs various improvements which are currently under evaluation.

References

Ahmad NR, Marks G, Mohiuddin M (1993) High-dose preoperative radiation for cancer of the rectum: impact of radiation dose on patterns of failure and survival. Int J Radiat Oncol Biol Phys 27:773–778

Berdov BA, Menteshashvili GZ (1990) Thermoradiotherapy of patients with locally advanced carcinoma of the rectum. Int J Hyperthermia 6:881–890

Chan A, Wong A, Langevin J, Khoo R (1993) Preoperative concurrent 5-fluorouracil infusion, mitomycin C and pelvic radiation therapy in tethered and fixed rectal carcinoma. Int J Radiat Oncol Biol Phys 25:791–799

Chen E, Mohiuddin M, Brodovsky H, Fishbein G, Marks G (1994) Downstaging of advanced rectal cancer following combined preoperative chemotherapy and high-dose radiation. Int J Radiat Oncol Biol Phys 30:169–175

Dahl O (1995) Interaction of heat and drugs in vitro and in vivo. In: Seegenschmiedt MH, Fessenden P, Vernon CC (eds) Principles and practice of thermotherapy and thermochemotherapy, vol 1: Biology, physiology, physics. Springer, Berlin Heidelberg New York, pp 103–121

Dewhirst MW (1995) Thermal dosimetry. In: Seegenschmiedt MH, Fessenden P, Vernon CC (eds) Principles and practice of thermoradiotherapy and thermochemotherapy, vol 1: Biology, physiology, physics. Springer Berlin Heidelberg New York, pp 123–136

Dosoretz DE, Gunderson LL, Hedberg S, Hoskins B, Blitzer PH, Shipley W, Cohen A (1983) Preoperative irradiation for unresectable rectal and rectosigmoid carcinomas. Cancer 52:814–818

Emami B, Pilepich M, Willett C, Munzenrider J, Miller HH (1982) Effect of preoperative irradiation on resectability of colorectal carcinomas. Int J Radiat Oncol Biol Phys 8:1295–1299

Gunderson LL, O'Connell MJ, Dozois RR (1992) The role of intra-operative irradiation in locally advanced primary and recurrent rectal adenocarcinoma. World J Surg 16:495–501

Hentschel M, Mirtsch S, Jordan A, Wust P, Vogl T, Semmler W, Wolf K-J, Felix R (1997) Heat response of HT29 cells depends strongly on perfusion: a 31 P NMR spectroscopy, HPLC and cell survival analysis. Int J Hyperthermia 13:69–82

Issels RD, Prenninger SW, Nagele A, Boehm E, Sauer H, Jauch K, Denecke H, Berger H, Peter K, Wilmanns W (1990) Ifosfamide plus etoposide combined with regional hyperthermia in patients with locally advanced sarcomas: a phase II study. J Clin Oncol 8:1818–1829

Jordan A, Scholz R, Schüler P, Wust P, Felix R (1987) Arrhenius analysis of the thermal response of human colonic adenocarcinoma cells in vitro using the multi-target, single-hit and the linear-quadratic model. Int J Hyperthermia 13:83–88

Konings AWT (1995) Interaction of heat and radiation in vitro and in vivo, In: Seegenschmiedt MH, Fessenden P, Vernon CC (eds) Principles and practice of thermotherapy and thermochemotherapy, vol. 1: Biology, physiology, physics. Springer Berlin Heidelberg New York pp 89-102

Leopold KA, Dewhirst MW, Samulski TV et al (1993) Cumulative minutes with T90 greater than TempIndex is predictive of response of superficial malignancies to hyperthermia and radiation. Int J Radiat Oncol Biol Phys 25:841-847

Minsky BD, Cohen AM, Kemeny N, Enker WE, Kelsen DP, Saltz L, Frankel J (1993) The efficacy of preoperative 5-fluorouracil, high-dose leucovorin, and sequential radiation therapy for unresectable rectal cancer. Cancer 71:3486-3492

Mohiuddin M, Ahmad NR, Marks G (1993) A selective approach to adjunctive therapy for cancer of the rectum. Int J Radiat Oncol Biol Phys 27:765-772

Mori M, Sugimachi K, Matsuda H, Ohno S, Inoue T et al (1989) Preoperative hyperthermochemotherapy for patients with rectal cancer. Dis Colon Rectum 32:316-322

Nadobny, J, Wust P, Seebass M, Deuflhard P, Felix R (1996) A volume-surface integral equation method for solving Maxwell's equations in electrically inhomogeneous media using tetrahedral grids. IEEE Trans Microwave Theor Tech 44:543-554

Oleson JR (1995) Hyperthermia from the clinic to the laboratory: a hypothesis. Int J Hyperthermia 11:315-322

Overgaard J (1989) The current and potential role of hyperthermia in radiotherapy. Int J Radiat Oncol Biol Phys 16:535-549

Overgaard J, Gonzalez Gonzalez D, Hume SP, Arcangeli G, Dahl O, Mella O, Bentzen SM (1995) Randomised trial of hyperthermia as adjuvant to radiotherapy for recurrent or metastatic malignant melanoma. Lancet 345:540-543

Perez CA, Gillespie B, Pajak T, Hornback NB, Emami B, Rubin P (1989) Quality assurance problems in clinical hyperthermia and their impact on therapeutic outcome: a report by the Radiation Therapy Oncology Group. Int J Radiat Oncol Biol Phys 16:551-558

Seebass M, Wust P, Gellermann J, Stalling D, Nadobny J, Felix R (1995) Dreidimensionale Simulation der nicht-invasiven Radiowellen-Hyperthermie. Minim Invasive Med 6:29-35

Streffer C (1995) Molecular and cellular mechanisms of hyperthermia. In: Seegenschmiedt MH, Fessenden P, Vernon CC (eds) Principles and practice of thermotherapy and thermochemotherapy, vol 1: Biology, physiology, physics. Springer, Berlin Heidelberg New York, pp 47-74

Valdagni R, Amichetti M (1993) Report of long-term follow-up in a randomized trial comparing radiation therapy and radiation therapy plus hyperthermia to metastatic lymphnodes in stage IV head and neck patients. Int J Radiat Oncol Biol Phys 28:163-169

Van der Zee J, Gonzalez Gonzalez D (1995) Hyperthermia in inoperable pelvic tumours. Strahlenther Onkol 171 (Sonderheft):1-56

Vernon CC, van der Zee J, Lui FF (1994) Collaborative phase III superficial hyperthermia trial. Joint Meeting of European Societies of Radiation Biology (ESRB) and Hyperthermic Oncology (ESHO), 1-4 June 1994, Amsterdam, Abstract Book, p 16

Wust P, Nadobny J, Seebass M, Dohlus M, John W, Felix R (1993) 3D-computation of E-fields by the volume-surface integral equation (VSIE) method in comparison to the finite-integration theory (FIT) method. IEEE Trans Biomed Eng 40:745-759

Wust P, Rau B, Gremmler M, Schlag P, Jordan A, Löffel J, Riess H, Felix R (1995) Radio-thermotherapy in multi-modal surgical treatment concepts. Onkologie 18:110-121

Wust P, Stahl H, Dieckmann K, Scheller S, Löffel J, Riess H, Jahnke V, Bier J, Felix R (1996a) Local hyperthermia of N2/N3 cervical lymphnode metastases: correlation of technical and thermal parameters with response. Int J Radiat Oncol Biol Phys 34:634-646

Wust P, Seebass M, Nadobny J, Deuflhard P, Mönich G, Felix R (1996b) Simulation studies promote technological development of radiofrequency hyperthermia. Int J Hyperthermia 12:477-494

You QS, Wang RZ, Suen GQ, Yan FC, Gao YJ, Cui SR, Zhao JH, Zhao TZ, Ding L (1993) Combination preoperative radiation and endocavitary hyperthermia for rectal cancer: long-term results of 44 patients. Int J Hyperthermia 9:19-24

Future Strategies to Improve Results of Therapy

Dietary and Chemopreventive Strategies

R. W. Owen

Division of Toxicology and Cancer Risk Factors, German Cancer Research Center, Im Neuenheimer Feld 280, 69120 Heidelberg, Germany

Abstract

Dietary and chemopreventive strategies may be used to stem the development of human cancer. This emerging field has increasing potential for influencing cancer incidence rates in defined high-risk groups and the general population. Colorectal cancer in particular, although the fourth most common cancer in the world, due to its temporal nature is amenable to both dietary and chemopreventive strategies. This chapter does not attempt to be all-embracing, but to serve its purpose will concentrate on major natural components of the diet and chemical additions that may be added to it, i.e. non-steroidal anti-inflammatory drugs, which by a common mechanism may reduce risk and recurrence of colorectal cancer.

Introduction

Colorectal cancer is a disease of affluent societies, and epidemiologic studies (Armstrong and Doll 1975; Willett et al. 1990; Giovanucci et al. 1994a, b) have clearly shown that dietary components are a major contributory factor. High consumption of fat and red meat are regarded as important in the promotion of the disease, perhaps through an additive effect on intestinal metabolism via increased hepatic secretion of biliary components and fermentation by the intestinal microflora (Hill et al. 1975; Reddy and Wynder 1977). By contrast, a high consumption of dietary fibre is regarded as ameliorative. Knowledge of the protective role of dietary fibre against colorectal cancer has its origins in the classic study of Burkitt (1971). This was based on epidemiologic studies in Africa which showed that a high intake of dietary fibre correlated strongly with high faecal weight. It was postulated that dietary fibre is protective against colorectal cancer by the simple mechanisms of stool bulking, acceleration of transit and dilution of potential endogenous carcinogens. This theory has recently received qualified support in the meta-analyses of Howe et al. (1992) and Cummings et al. (1992).

These basic observations, however, which have their origins in the late 1960s, are after more than 30 years of research still not clearly resolved. Research into the role of fat, bile acids and fibre in colorectal cancer goes on virtually unabated with slight variations of the themes, but still the discovery of a definitive proximate carcinogen produced in the colorectum either from the diet or the environment is awaited. Despite this, with a considerable expansion of horizons it is obvious that progress is being made, especially in the areas of genetic susceptibility, polymorphisms and DNA adduct research. Nevertheless, it is not the intention to cover these rapidly expanding areas here; rather, a format akin to metabolic epidemiology will be addressed, with special emphasis on the bile acids, calcium, phytic acid, non-steroidal anti-inflammatory drugs and reactive oxygen species and their role in dietary and chemopreventive strategies.

Bile Acids

The notion that bile acid metabolites may be involved in the aetiology of colorectal cancer dates back to keynote publications early in the 1970s. The principal hypotheses (Hill et al. 1971; Reddy and Wynder 1973), based largely on epidemiologic data, were that high dietary intakes of animal fat (common in western countries) elicited a response within the intestinal hepatic circulation to produce greater quantities of bile acids to aid the digestive process. As a result of an increased proportional loss of these bile acids to the large bowel, and metabolism by the indigenous microflora, an increase in cytotoxic secondary bile acids might be expected to occur in the intestinal lumen. These hypotheses were vindicated by the data of Hill et al. (1975) and Reddy and Wynder (1977), who showed that colorectal cancer patients in England and the USA respectively excreted significantly elevated levels of faecal secondary bile acids. In the following 15 years support was gained from both in vitro (Silverman and Andrews 1977; Wilpart et al. 1983) and animal model (Narisawa et al. 1974; Galloway et al. 1986) experiments showing both a co-carcinogenic and promotional effect of these substances on colorectal neoplasia. The hypotheses were nevertheless considered controversial because of a number of contradictory case-control studies (Moskowitz et al. 1979; Mudd et al. 1980; Murray et al. 1980), but they led to a further plausible explanation of how the incidence of colorectal cancer could be modulated by dietary intervention with calcium.

Calcium

Over the last decade there has been considerable interest in the study of calcium as a chemopreventive agent against colorectal cancer. The interest stems from epidemiological studies (Garland et al. 1985; Sorenson et al. 1988) which show that the incidence of the disease is lower in regions of western industrialized societies where the consumption of calcium-containing dietary constituents such as dairy products is relatively high. A hypothesis was first mooted by Newmark et al. (1984) based on the considerations that the consumption of calcium leads to a higher concentration of this ion in the intestinal lumen, which reacts with endogenous secretions of the liver – namely the bile acids – and also dietary long-chain fatty acids to form insoluble complexes, thereby nullifying the purported cytotoxic effects of these lipids. This hypothesis was also based on several experimental animal studies (Wargovich et al. 1983, 1984) which showed that calcium can ameliorate the damaging effects of these agents when it is applied intracolonically and was supported by later animal studies investigating the role of calcium in preventing the cytotoxic effect of intestinal lipids and thereby influencing the development of colorectal cancer (Bird et al. 1986; Rafter et al. 1986).

These studies were followed by calcium intervention trials in humans but the results overall have been equivocal. Several studies (Lipkin et al. 1989; Rozen et al. 1989; Steinbach et al. 1994) have shown that supplementing the human diet with calcium can reduce intestinal cell proliferation, an intermediate biomarker of colorectal cancer; others (Gregoire et al. 1989; Stern et al. 1990) have shown no effect, whilst one (Kleibeuker et al. 1993) has shown the opposite.

In addition to the hypothetical and intervention considerations, Van der Meer and De Vries (1985) have provided a plausible molecular mechanism in vitro to explain how calcium may mediate its effects; the message conveyed from a series of in vivo studies (Govers and Van der Meer 1993; Lapre et al. 1993; Welberg et al. 1993) is that calcium intervention leads to a significant reduction in cell proliferation, and the mechanism is clear: 'supplementary dietary calcium stimulates the formation of insoluble calcium phosphate in the intestine, which results in increased binding of cytotoxic luminal bile acids.' Furthermore, Van der Meer et al. (1990) have suggested that the amount of bile acid associated with calcium can be determined by the resolubilisation of calcium soaps with ethylenediaminetetraacetic acid (EDTA). The rationale indicated, is that because EDTA is a potent chelator of divalent cations, especially calcium, incubation of faeces in the presence of EDTA will solubilise those bile acids complexed to calcium.

The theoretical and molecular mechanisms put forward to explain the protective effect of calcium against colorectal cancer appear to be flawed however. This is exemplified by a recent study (Owen et al. 1995) which shows, using organically synthesised calcium soaps of the bile acids, that the EDTA method described to account for the appreciable levels of calcium bile acid soaps in faeces gives almost identical results for free bile acids (Fig. 1a) and calcium-bound bile acids (Fig. 1b), in that both are solubilised to a similar extent and that the solubilisation of faecal bile acids by this method is significantly dependent on both total and primary bile acid concentration.

In consideration of the equivocal clinical data mentioned above, a long-term, double-blind intervention trial was undertaken by Weisgerber et al. (1996) in polypectomised sporadic adenoma patients, in whom the putative

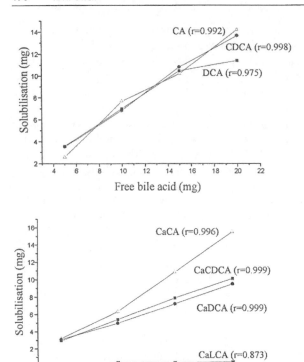

Fig. 1. a Solubilisation of free bile acids by tris/EDTA. CA, Cholic acid; CDCA, chenodeoxycholic acid; DCA, deoxycholic acid. **b** Solubilisation of Calcium bile acid soaps by tris/EDTA. CaCA, calcium cholate; CaCDCA, calcium chenodeoxycholate; CaDCA, calcium deoxycholate; CaLCA, calcium lithocholate

role of calcium (2 g/day) as a protective factor in colonic carcinogenesis was studied. The results show that despite differences in stool biochemistry elicited by supplementary calcium, after 9 months' intervention a similar non-significant decrease of total proliferation index (PI%) in sigmoidal mucosa was evident in both the calcium (13.5–11.4) and placebo groups (13.7–10.7).

An increase in the concentration and daily excretion of total bile acids, primary bile acids, long-chain fatty acids and long-chain fatty acid soaps was also observed in the calcium group, whilst there was no significant reduction in the concentration of the potentially toxic free bile acids and long-chain fatty acids. The conclusions that can be drawn from the measurement of cell proliferation and faecal characteristics in this group of patients is that calcium is unlikely to be of use as a chemopreventive agent against colorectal cancer in compromised subjects.

There may be several reasons why intervention with dietary calcium gives conflicting results. The capacity of calcium to reduce cell proliferation may be short-term and only a transient effect is observed prior to intestinal adaptation. This would explain why most short-term studies show it to be effective and long-term studies do not. In the absence of short-term placebo-controlled trials it is probable that the apparent positive results with calcium are a result of inappropriate study design. An appropriate study design is essential in calcium intervention trials, especially in adenoma patients who have undergone polypectomy, because it has been shown that a significant temporal decrease in colonic cell proliferation occurs in adenoma-free colons over a 2-year period (Risio et al. 1991). This observation may explain why calcium intervention in polypectomised patients without a placebo-control group appears effective.

Alternatively, calcium may exert its effect only in younger people who are able to maintain or enhance the calcium gradient within the mucosal crypt and colonocytes, thereby facilitating differentiation and apoptosis as described by Whitfield (1992). That the Whitfield model only applies to younger people is supported by the data of Weisgerber et al. (1996) on relatively elderly people. At entry to the study, the mean PI% of all the patients was significantly positively associated with soluble calcium in faeces. After intervention PI% was decreased in both the calcium and placebo groups to a similar extent despite a significant increase in faecal-soluble calcium in the former group. This is again at odds with the Whitfield model, and because increased cell proliferation also positively correlated with patient age, it indicates that high luminal calcium concentration as mentioned above may only be effective in reducing cell proliferation in younger people who are able to maintain the necessary calcium gradient that stimulates differentiation and apoptosis.

These conclusions are further supported by the findings on calcium balance in the study group. At entry to the study dietary intake of calcium by the patient group as a whole was over 900 mg/day. Under these conditions obligatory renal loss of calcium (which reflects absorption capacity) was only 86 mg/day, compared to an expected 155 mg/day. This represents an almost 100% decrease in absorption of calcium, and dietary supplementation with 2 g/day calcium had little effect on urinary loss. According to the Whitfield model, therefore, an increase in soluble calcium would be of no benefit if intestinal transmembrane reflux of calcium is diminished in older people. This appears to be the case here and is probably a valid reason why calcium intervention was no more effective in lowering PI% than placebo. This has support in that decreased calcium absorption with increased age is a well-recognised phenomenon and may be one general reason why elderly patients exhibit a higher proliferative activity in the colonic epithelium than younger people.

Because calcium absorption in the large intestine is dependent on the supply of itamin D and is stimulated by the active form of this vitamin, it may be prudent in future studies with elderly people to incorporate this vitamin into the intervention protocol. This may re-establish the ability of colonocytes to maintain a positive calcium gradient and effectively reduce cell proliferation.

The results also indicate that calcium does not operate via an indirect antitropic effect in older patients, because the calcium balance data show that calcium absorption was severely impaired and therefore an effective gradient in the colonocytes could not be maintained. This is probably an age-related phenomenon and indicates that calcium supplementation is unlikely to be of major therapeutic use in the reduction of cell proliferation and adenoma recurrence in elderly people. Furthermore, perhaps it is expecting too much of calcium to behave as a chemotherapeutic agent in adenoma patients, and future studies should concentrate on calcium intervention as a means of chemoprevention in healthy high-risk populations. The data from the ongoing pan-European calcium/fibre intervention study in sporadic adenoma patients ($n=>700$) should help to clarify this situation (Faivre et al. 1991).

Phytic Acid

The protective effect ascribed to fibre has been fortified by a range of diverse epidemiologic and animal experiments, but it has been suggested by Graf and Eaton (1985), prompted by certain inconsistencies in the dietary fibre data, that it is the phytic acid content which is the most crucial ingredient. Phytic acid, a hexaphosphorylated sugar, is a ubiquitous plant component that may constitute 1%–5% by weight of most cereals, nuts, legumes and oil seeds (Maga 1982). The antioxidative properties of phytic acid are ascribed to its chelating potential. Phytic acid exhibits a high affinity for all polyvalent cations; metal phytate complexes are well known to be insoluble over a wide pH range, and this is particularly true for iron-phytate chelates. For this reason Graf and Eaton (1990) postulate that all of the antioxidant properties of phytic acid derive from its relatively high binding affinity for iron. Iron-catalysed reactions play a crucial role in oxidative damage to biological materials and can be generated by a combination of two commonly described mechanisms, namely the Haber-Weiss and Fenton reactions as shown below:

Fe^{3+}-chelate + $O_2^{\bullet-}$ → O_2 + Fe^{2+}-chelate

Fe^{2+}-chelate + H_2O_2 → Fe^{3+}-chelate + $OH^{\bullet}$ + OH^-

Net reaction: $O_2^{\bullet-}$ + H_2O_2 → O_2 + $OH^{\bullet}$ + OH^-

Since the keynote publication of Graf and Eaton (1985) the influence that phytic acid may have in the genesis of colorectal cancer has received substantial support from animal model studies (Nielson et al. 1987; Nelson et al. 1989; Ullah and Shamsuddin 1990). Further support for the hypothesis of Graf and Eaton (1990) comes from studies on iron status and risk of cancer in humans. Stevens et al. (1988) reported that increased body iron stores were significantly associated with colon cancer in a national survey (NHANES 1), and this has been supported by a recent case control study

(Nelson et al. 1994) showing that adenoma risk is positively associated with elevated serum ferritin levels.

Despite all the circumstantial evidence, however, until recently no study had been conducted in the clinical domain to bring together the various factors of the phytic acid/reactive oxygen species hypothesis (Graf and Eaton 1990) and its implications for cancer. To test whether or not this hypothesis has relevance in humans, a high-performance liquid chromatography (HPLC) system has been developed by Owen et al. (1996a) and utilized for the analysis of phytic acid in selected foods and human faeces. Cell proliferation rate and faecal lipid, mineral and phytic acid content of patients with sporadic adenomatous polyps have been measured (Weisgerber et al. 1996) to establish any interrelation which may have a bearing on the aetiology of colorectal cancer.

Analysis of phytic acid in selected foodstuffs showed a good correlation with other methods in that the highest phytic acid content of those compared was found in wheat bran and the lowest in soy beans. Phytic acid levels were also determined in foodstuffs which have not been previously reported and of these coriander, tomato and green pepper seeds were found to contain appreciable amounts (Table 1) (Owen at al. 1996a).

The HPLC method was also found to be appropriate for the measurement of phytic acid in human faeces. Phytic acid was detected in faecal extracts of the adenoma patients in the range 0.68–4.00 µmol/g wet faeces and 55–2038 µmol/day. Linear regression analyses of phytic acid versus faecal lipid and mineral content and intestinal cell proliferation showed that the amount of phytic acid in the stool was strongly correlated (Fig. 2a) with faecal iron ($r=0.52$; $p=0.00004$), unsaturated fatty acids ($r=0.35$; $p=0.004$) and total

Table 1. Phytic acid (%, dry weight) content of a range of foods

Food sample	External standard[a]			Literature values
	Phytic acid	Sodium phytate	Sodium phytate[b]	
Sesame seeds	2.21±0.02	7.83±0.07	5.56±0.05	5.36±0.09
Wheat bran	2.28±0.08	8.14±0.37	5.78±0.22	5.03±1.85
Peanuts	0.86±0.02	3.05±0.07	2.17±0.04	1.88±0.05
Soy beans	0.89±0.06	3.09±0.22	2.20±0.16	1.84±0.03
Tomato seeds	1.24±0.14	4.36±0.49	3.10±0.35	np
Chilli seeds	0.56±0.06	1.90±0.21	1.34±0.15	np
Coriander seeds	1.11±0.03	3.93±0.10	2.79±0.07	np
Pepper seeds	0.57±0.01	1.96±0.04	1.39±0.03	np
Millett	0.18±0.01	0.62±0.03	0.44±0.02	np

Data from Owen et al. (1996b).

np, Not published.

[a] Results expressed as % (mean±SD) of 2–4 samples: lyophilised, pulverised and defatted with pentane (not corrected for defatting).

[b] Sodium phytate corrected for salt content.

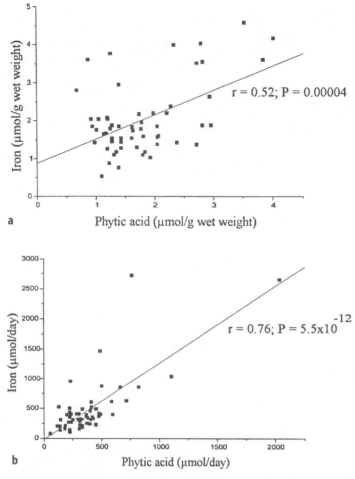

Fig. 2. a Relation between faecal iron and phytic acid concentration in adenoma patients. **b** Relation between daily faecal iron excretion and phytic acid concentration in adenoma patients

calcium content of the stool ($r=0.34$; $p=0.01$). The association between phytic acid and minerals was even stronger when analysed on a daily basis: phytic acid versus iron, $r=0.76$; $p=5.5\times10^{-12}$ (Fig. 2b): phytic acid versus total calcium, $r=0.59$; $p=1.36\times10^{-6}$.

This study shows clearly for the first time that a strong association exists between the presence of phytic acid and iron in the large intestine of humans as evaluated by faecal biochemistry. High concentrations of phytic acid chelate intestinal iron thereby preventing it from partaking in the generation of reactive oxygen species (ROS) which may damage DNA, leading to mutation and cancer. The sequestration of iron in this way may also lower absorption and prevent excessive accumulation of body iron stores, which is also associated with colorectal cancer. Further population, case control and clinical trials are warranted in this area to fully evaluate the chemopreventive potential of phytic acid.

Non-steroidal anti-inflammatory Drugs

Non-steroidal anti-inflammatory drugs (NSAIDs) are believed to mediate their effects in colorectal neoplasia by altered metabolism of arachidonic acid via inhibition of cyclooxygenase (COX) enzymes, thereby reducing the production of prostaglandins, prostacyclin and thromboxanes. It is now known that two forms of COX enzymes exist, COX-1 and COX-2 (Marnett 1992). COX-1 is expressed in most tissues and is thought to be the product of a constitutively expressed gene (O'Neil and Ford-Hutchinson 1993). It is involved in cellular homeostasis, synthesising prostaglandins in response to physiological stimuli at a rate proportional to the availability of the substrate arachidonic acid. Prostaglandins in the gastrointestinal tract have an important protective role in the maintenance of microvascular integrity, the regulation of cell division and the production of mucus. COX-2, on the other hand, has been shown to be inducible (Dubois et al. 1994) in non-transformed rat intestinal epithelial cells in vitro by growth factors and tumour promoters at sites of inflammation. Macrophages and other inflammatory cells have abundant COX-2 activity. Levels of COX-2 are also increased several-fold in 90% of human colorectal carcinomas and 40% of colorectal adenomas, and therefore the products of COX-2 may drive inflammatory processes and carcinogenesis (Eberhart et al. 1994). Quite recently it has been shown that the recombinant COX-2 enzyme has a different sensitivity to NSAID inhibition than COX-1 (Meade et al. 1993). Therefore it is possible that the COX enzymes have different modalities with respect to colorectal neoplasia, and the development of NSAIDs which are specific inhibitors of COX-2 may be an important landmark in the already vast potential for NSAIDs in the prevention of colorectal cancer. However, despite this there is a growing literature on two NSAIDs in particular, aspirin and sulindac, which appear to be extremely promising as chemopreventive agents although they both preferentially inhibit the COX-1 enzyme over COX-2.

Epidemiologic case control and cohort studies suggest that the use of aspirin is associated with an approximately 50% reduction in the development of colorectal cancer. The data for humans have recently been reviewed by Little (1994) and in this report three of four cohort and three case control studies showed an inverse relation with the use of aspirin. Similar associations were also described in three studies of aspirin use and the incidence of colorectal polyps. In this review it was also noted, however, that in the one available randomised trial no protective effect of low-dose aspirin (325 mg) taken every other day against invasive colorectal cancer or colorectal polyps was found. Since this publication a further prospective cohort study has been described (Giovanucci et al. 1994b). The setting of this study was male health professionals throughout the USA, 47 900 of whom responded to a mailed questionnaire. Regular users of aspirin (at least=twice/week) had a significantly lower risk of total colorectal cancer (relative risk=0.68; 95% CI, 0.52-0.92) and advanced metastatic and total colorectal cancer (RR=0.51; CI, 0.32-0.84) after controlling for confounding variables such as age, history of polyp, previous endoscopy, parenteral history of colorectal cancer, smoking, history of polyp, body mass, physical activity, and intake of red meat, vitamin E and alcohol. This well-designed study is impressive evidence for the protective effects of aspirin against colorectal cancer.

Sulindac on the other hand, unlike aspirin, is not available for general prescription and has been utilised predominantly for the treatment of colorectal adenomatous polyps in patients with familial adenomatous polyposis (FAP). This is an autosomal dominant disorder the hallmark of which is the development of hundreds to thousands of colorectal polyps in adults, usually below the age of 30. The pioneers of sulindac use for the regression of colorectal polyps were Waddell and Loughry (1983), and since then a number of groups have reported the daily administration of 150-400 mg/day sulindac with varying degrees of success. To date the most impressive data have been reported by Winde et al. (1995) in whose study, by contrast to previous ones, low-dose sulindac maintenance therapy was given intrarectally instead of by the oral route.

Twenty-five patients with histologically confirmed FAP were entered into the study at least 3 years after colectomy with ileorectal anastomosis. Fifteen of these served as the study group and 10 as a non-randomised control group. At entry sulindac suppositories (150 mg) were administred twice daily for 6 weeks, and thereafter on visible reduction in the number of polyps by endoscopy the daily dose of sulindac was lowered sequentially. The data from this group show that the number of polyps was reduced significantly during sulindac therapy. In the study group, after treatment with sulindac (300 mg/day) for 6 weeks the number of polyps (Σ 208) was reduced by 83% (Σ 36) and thereafter by 96% after 18 weeks (Σ 8) such that no polyps were visible after 24 weeks. The number of polyps in the control group remained relatively constant during this period (initial, Σ 99: final, Σ 92). Furthermore, no relapse of polyps was observed after 132 weeks during which the average daily dose of sulindac was reduced significantly from 300 to 67 mg/day (Table 2). Clearly, in FAP patients the administration of sulindac as a low-dose suppository in the rectum is an unmitigated success in the eradication of polyps, and further reports from this group will be eagerly awaited.

It is interesting to note the varying degrees of success between the use of sulindac in FAP patients an in those with sporadic polyps. To date there are only two reports for comparison. In one small study (Hixson et al. 1993) involving five patients, only one patient had partial regression of a polyp after 3 months of sulindac treatment. In the other, very recent double-blind placebo-controlled study, the effect of sulindac (300 mg/day) for 4 months was compared in 44 patients (22 cases, 22 controls) with sporadic adenoma (Ladenheim et al. 1995). Using an intention to treat analysis, the data showed that five patients (23%) receiving sulindac and three subjects receiving place-

Table 2. Regression of the total number of polyps and of flat mucosa elevations in familial polyposis patients in relation to sulindac treatment over 132 weeks

Study group				Control group
Control intervals	Treatment mean dose/day (mg)	Polyps Σ (n)	Flat mucosal elevations	Polyps Σ (n)
U0	0	208	–	99
U6	300.0	36	3	–
U12	220.0	33	3	103
U18	170.0	8	3	–
U24	120.0	–	2	92
U30	73.3	–	2	–
U36	50.0	–	6	87
U42	53.5	–	5	–
U48	53.3	–	5	85
U60	70.0	–	1	88
U72	83.3	–	3	78
U84	76.6	–	1	86
U96	70.0	–	0	88
U108	66.6	–	0	84
U120	66.6	–	1	95
U132	66.6	–	2	92

Data from Winde et al. (1995).
U, Re-examination after n weeks

bo had complete regression of their polyps after 4 months. When this was based on adenomatous polyps, 5 of 14 patients (36%) taking sulindac and 3 of 15 (20%) taking placebo had adenoma regression. By neither analysis were the differences significant, however. The authors conclude it is unlikely that the rate of regression of polyps in sporadic adenoma patients on sulindac therapy is 50% or more.

Taking these two studies together it is obvious that there is a paucity of data regarding the modality of sulindac for the treatment of sporadic polyps and that rectal suppositories are far more effective in FAP patients than the oral route. This may also apply in the treatment of sporadic adenoma. Therefore further studies are recommended in FAP patients to ascertain whether the data of Winde et al. (1995) can be reproduced, and it would be of great interest if such a regime used by this group was also applied to patients with sporadic adenoma.

Reactive Oxygen Species

An alternative explanation for the efficiency of NSAIDs in the prevention of colorectal cancer is their undoubted ability to scavenge ROS. This is emphasised in a recent study (Owen et al. 1996b) in which salicylic acid, the active component of aspirin, was used as a sink to detect the formation of the hydroxyl radical, a potent DNA-damaging species.

ROS such as superoxide anion ($O_2^{\bullet-}$) and the hydroxyl radical (OH$^\bullet$) and the non-radical hydrogen peroxide (H_2O_2) are possibly involved in a range of human diseases, namely atherosclerosis, ischaemia/reperfusion injury, rheumatoid arthritis, inflammatory bowel disease, oral cancer and colorectal cancer. Of the ROS spectrum OH$^\bullet$ appears to be particularly dangerous due to its rapid and non-specific reactivity with most biomolecules, A mechanism which has been described for the formation of OH$^\bullet$ in biological systems is a combination of the Haber-Weiss and Fenton reactions, as mentioned earlier.

In view of the increasing interest in ROS as aetiologic agents in human disease, and a growing literature (Logan et al. 1993; Little 1994; Paganini-Hill 1994) on aspirin as a possible chemopreventive agent against colorectal cancer, an HPLC method based on ion-pair chromatography was developed to study the generation of ROS in vitro. The method, using salicylic acid as an aromatic probe, enables the kinetics of ROS production in model systems such as the hypoxanthine/xanthine oxidase system and by faecal bacteria to be studied in detail and is therefore of particular relevance to colorectal cancer. The HPLC method is ideal for monitoring the dynamics of both the hypoxanthine/xanthine oxidase system and the hydroxylation of salicylic acid by OH$^\bullet$ in this model system. Utilising an aqueous mobile phase (pH 4.3) containing the ion-pair reagent tetrabutylammonium hydroxide (0.005 M), baseline separation of hypoxanthine (9.0 min) and its hydroxylated products xanthine (10.3 min) and uric acid (12.4 min) was effected (Fig. 3a). Furthermore the incorporation of methanol (40%) in this mobile phase facilitates the separation (Fig. 3b) of 2,5-dihydroxy benzoic acid (4.2 min) and 2,3-dihydroxy benzoic acid (4.6 min), the products of OH$^\bullet$ attack on salicylic acid (7.00 min).

The method has been validated by incorporation of various classical reagents used to authenticate the generation of ROS in biological systems. Addition of free-radical scavengers such as butanol, dimethyl sulphoxide (DMSO), ethanol and mannitol reduced diphenol production in a dose-dependent manner (Fig. 4). Scavenging potency was of the order DMSO > butanol > ethanol > mannitol. Addition of the enzyme inhibitors catalase and superoxide dismutase (SOD) also severely curtailed OH$^\bullet$ production in a dose-dependent manner (Fig. 5).

Because phytic acid has been mooted (Graf and Eaton 1990) as an important constituent of dietary fibre with regard to its protective effect against colorectal cancer, this hexaphosphorylated sugar was also tested in the system. While free-radical scavengers in the mM range were required to inhibit OH$^\bullet$ attack on salicylic acid in the current system, the concentration of free phy-

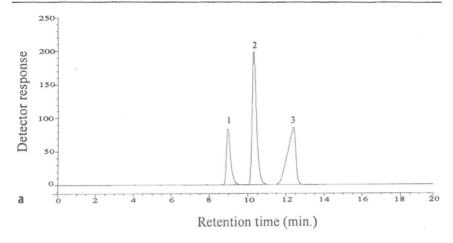

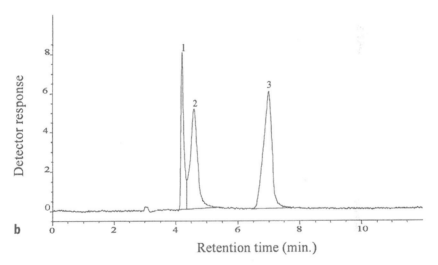

Fig. 3. a HPLC chromatogram of hypoxanthine and its hydroxylated products xanthine and uric acid. *Peak 1:* Hypoxanthine (retention time = 9.0 min); *peak 2:* xanthine (retention time = 10.3 min); *peak 3:* uric acid (retention time = 12.4 min). **b** HPLC chromatogram of salicylic acid and its hydroxylated products 2,3-dihydroxy benzoic acid and 2,5-dihydroxy benzoic acid. *Peak 1:* 2,5-dihydroxy benzoic acid (retention time = 4.2 min); *peak 2:* 2,3-dihydroxy benzoic acid (retention time = 4.6 min); *peak 3:* salicylic acid (retention time = 7.0 min)

tic acid and sodium phytate required was an order of magnitude less in an EDTA-deplete system: phytic acid and sodium phytate in the range 50-2000 µM reduced diphenol production in a dose-dependent manner (Fig. 6).

This new HPLC method has been applied to the evaluation of ROS generation by faecal bacteria and shows that 1:100 dilutions of faecal bacteria obtained from stool samples of adenoma patients (Weisgerber et al. 1996) are capable of generating significant quantities of ROS as evinced by the production of diphenols from salicylic acid. This supports the previous observation

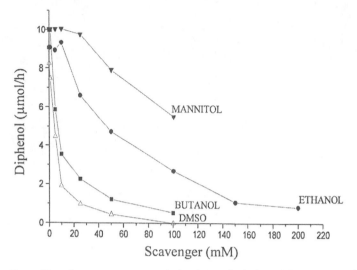

Fig. 4. Effect of various scavengers on hydroxylation of salicylic acid. Data represent the mean of duplicate experiments

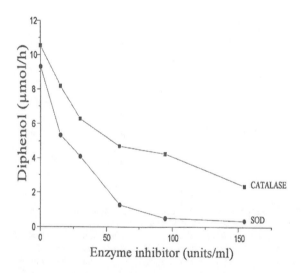

Fig. 5. Effect of enzyme inhibitors on hydroxylation of salicylic acid. Data represent the mean of duplicate experiments

of Babbs (1990). In ten samples studied thus far, faecal dilutions, albeit in a favourable aerobic environment with glucose as carbon source, produced on average 0.35 mM diphenol/g wet faeces after 18 h incubation at 37 °C (Table 3). The extent of OH• generation in these human faecal samples is approximately 200-fold higher than that reported for rat faeces (Babbs 1990). There-

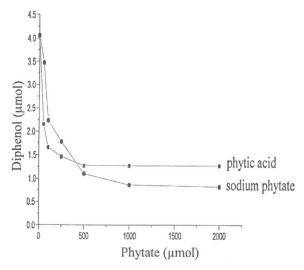

Fig. 6. Effect of phytate on hydroxylation of salicylic acid in an EDTA-deplete system. Data represent the mean of duplicate experiments

Table 3. Hydroxylation of salicylic acid by human faecal samples as determined by HPLC

Sample number	Faecal wet weight (g)	Diphenol produced[a] mM/g	mM/day
1	240	0.195	46.8
2	153	0.358	54.77
3	389	0.131	50.96
4	122	0.414	50.51
5	220	0.495	92.62
6	198	0.377	74.65
7	362	0.191	69.14
8	167	0.377	62.96
9	341	0.436	148.68
10	242	0.555	134.31
Mean±SEM	243±129	0.35±0.04	78.5±11.4

Data from Owen et al. (1996b).

[a] Results expressed as mean±SEM of duplicate experiments. Hydroxylation of salicylic acid was determined by HPLC.

fore the capacity for the generation of ROS by the human faecal flora in vitro appears to be an easily detectable phenomenon, but it obviously cannot be fully extrapolated to the in vivo situation within the large intestine where anaerobiosis predominates.

Nevertheless studies are underway to evaluate the effect of different dietary regimens on the potential of the bacterial flora to generate ROS in the clinical situation and animal model systems. The role of phytic acid and NSAIDs in particular is being addressed using DNA adducts as the intermediate endpoint for colorectal cancer, and this should help to clarify the involvement of ROS in the aetiology of this disease.

Conclusions

The conclusions that can be drawn from the subject content of this chapter, which spans almost 30 years of research, is that colorectal cancer is readily amenable to both dietary and chemopreventive strategies. The early work which focused on macrocomponents of the diet, namely fat and fibre, although lacking support from actual proven mechanisms, may still be relevant in terms of general recommendations to the public, in that a significant reduction in the incidence of this disease would obviously accrue if the fat content of the diet was restricted to no more than 30% and fibre intake increased to at least 30 g/day.

It is the opinion of the author that such recommendations would be of little use to the surgeon in the prevention of recurrent cancer after major surgery however. While such approaches would be prudent, the administration of drugs of the NSAID class, especially sulindac, may be a better choice in reducing the need for further surgery. The NSAID's including aspirin and perhaps phytic acid also appear to have potential in both primary and secondary prevention terms in high-risk groups. The utility of these compounds can be further enhanced by a more complete understanding of their mechanisms of action. This will no doubt be forthcoming in the near future and therefore provides grounds for optimism that the incidence and mortality of colorectal cancer can be severely reduced in the coming years.

References

Armstrong B, Doll R (1975) Environmental factors and cancer incidence and mortality in different countries, with special reference to dietary practices. Int J Cancer 15:617–631

Babbs CF (1990) Free radicals and the etiology of colon cancer. Free Radic Biol Med 8:191–200

Bird RP, Schneider R, Stamp D, Bruce WR (1986) Effect of dietary calcium and cholic acid on the proliferative indices of murine colonic epithelium. Carcinogenesis 7:1657–1661

Burkitt DP (1971) Epidemiology of cancer of the colon and rectum. Cancer 28:3–13

Cummings JH, Bingham SA, Heaton KW, Eastwood MA (1992) Faecal weight, colon cancer risk and dietary intake of nonstarch polysaccharides (dietary fiber). Gastroenterology 103:1783–1789

Dubois RN, Awad J, Morrow J, Roberts LJ, Bishop PR (1994) Regulation of eicosanoid production and mitogenesis in rat intestinal epithelial cells by transforming growth factor-α and phorbol ester. J Clin Invest 93:493–498

Eberhart CE, Coffey RJ, Radhika A, Giardiello FM, Ferrenbach S, Dubois RN (1994) Upregulation of cyclooxygenase-2 gene expression in human colorectal adenomas and adenocarcinomas. Gastroenterology 107:1183–1188

Faivre J, Doyon F, Boutron MC (1991) The ECP calcium fibre polyp prevention study. The ECP Colon Group. Eur J Cancer Prev 1 (Suppl 2):83-89

Galloway DJ, Owen RW, Jarrett F, Boyle P, Hill MJ, George WD (1986) Experimental colorectal cancer: the relationship of diet and faecal bile acid concentration to tumour induction. Br J Surg 73:233-237

Garland CF, Barrett-Connor E, Rossof AH, Shekelle RB, Criqui MH, Paul O (1985) Dietary vitamin D and calcium and risk of colorectal cancer: a 19-year prospective study in men. Lancet i:307-309

Giovanucci E, Rimm EB, Stampfer MJ, Colditz GA, Ascherio A, Willett WC (1994a) Intake of fat, meat and fiber in relation to risk of colon cancer in men. Cancer Res 54:2390-2397

Giovanucci E, Rimm EB, Stampfer MJ, Colditz GA, Ascherio A, Willett WC (1994b) Aspirin use and the risk of colorectal cancer and adenoma in male health professionals. Ann Intern Med 121:241-246

Govers MJ, Van der Meer R (1993) Effects of dietary calcium and phosphate on the intestinal interactions between calcium, phosphate, fatty acids and bile acids. Gut 34:365-370

Graf E, Eaton JW (1985) Dietary suppression of colonic cancer. Fiber or phytate? Cancer 56:717-718

Graf E, Eaton JW (1990) Antioxidant functions of phytic acid. Free Radic Biol Med 8:61-69

Gregoire RC, Stern HS, Yeung KS, Stadler J, Langley S, Furrer R, Bruce WR (1989) Effect of calcium supplementation on mucosal cell proliferation in high risk patients for colon cancer. Gut 30:376-382

Hallyer J, Bjarnason I (1995) NSAIDs, COX-2 inhibitors, and the gut. Lancet 346:520-522

Hill MJ, Drasar BS, Aries VC, Crowther JS, Hawksworth GM, Williams REO (1971) Bacteria and the aetiology of large bowel cancer. Lancet i:95-100

Hill MJ, Drasar BS, Williams REO, Meade TW, Cox AG, Simpson JEP, Morson BC (1975) Faecal bile acids and clostridia in patients with cancer of the large bowel. Lancet i:535-539

Hixson LJ, Earnest DL, Fennerty MB, Sampliner RE (1993) NSAID effect on sporadic colon polyps. Am J Gastroenterol 10:1647-1649

Howe GR, Benito E, Castelleto R, Cornee J, Esteve J, Gallagher RP, Iscovich JM, Deng-ao J, Kaaks R, Kune GA, Kune S, L'Abbe KA, Lee HP, Lee M, Miller AB, Peters RK, Potter JD, Riboli E, Slattery ML, Trichopoulos D, Tuyns A, Tzonou A, Whittemore AS, Wu-Williams AH, Shu Z (1992) Dietary intake of fiber and decreased risk of cancers of the colon and rectum: evidence from the combined analysis of 13 case-control studies. J Natl Cancer Inst 84:1887-1896

Kleibeuker JH, Welberg JWM, Mulder NH, Van der Meer R, Cats A, Limburg AJ, Kreumer WMT, Hardonk MJ, De Vries EG (1993) Epithelial cell proliferation in the sigmoid colon of patients with adenomatous polyps increases during oral calcium supplementation. Br J Cancer 67:500-503

Ladenheim J, Garcia G, Titzer D, Herzenberg H, Lavori P, Edson R, Omary MB (1995) Effect of sulindac on sporadic colonic polyps. Gastroenterology 108:1083-1087

Lapre JA, De Vries HT, Termont DS, Kleibeuker JH, De Vries EG, Van der Meer R (1993) Mechanism of the protective effect of supplementary dietary calcium on cytolytic activity of fecal water. Cancer Res 53:248-253

Lipkin M, Friedman E, Winawer SJ, Newmark H (1989) Colonic epithelial cell proliferation in responders and nonresponders to supplementary dietary calcium. Cancer Res 29:248-254

Little J (1994) Aspirin and other nonsteroidal anti-inflammatory drugs and colorectal neoplasia. Int J Oncol 5:1151-1162

Logan RF, Little J, Hawtin PG, Hardcastle JD (1993) Effect of aspirin and non-steroidal anti-inflammatory drugs on colorectal adenomas: case-control study of subjects participating in the Nottingham faecal occult blood screening programme. B Med J 307:285-289

Maga JA (1982) Phytate; its chemistry, occurrence, food interactions, nutritional significance and methods of analysis. J Agric Food Chem 30:1-9

Marnett LJ (1992) Aspirin and the potential role of prostaglandins in colon cancer. Cancer Res 52:5575-5589

Meade EA, Smith WL, DeWitt DL (1993) Differential endoperoxide synthase (cyclooxygenase) isozymes by aspirin and other non-steroidal anti-inflammatory drugs. J Biol Chem 268:6610–6614

Moskowitz M, White C, Barnett RN, Stevens S, Russell E, Vargo D, Floch MH (1979) Diet, fecal bile acids and neutral sterols in carcinoma of the colon. Dig Dis Sci 24:746–751

Mudd DG, McKelvey STD, Norwood W, Elmore DT, Roy AD (1980) Faecal bile acid concentrations of patients with carcinoma or increased risk of carcinoma in the large bowel. Gut 21:587–590

Murray WR, Blackwood A, Trotter JM, Calman KC, Mackay C (1980) Faecal bile acids and clostridia in the aetiology of colorectal cancer. Br J Cancer 41:923–928

Narisawa T, Magadia NE, Weisberger JH, Wynder EL (1974) Promoting effects of bile acids on colon carcinogenesis after intrarectal instillation of N-methyl-N[1]-nitrosoguanidine in rats. J Natl Cancer Inst 53:1093–1097

Nelson RL, Yoo SJ, Tanure JC, Andrianopoulos S, Misumi A (1989) The effect of iron on experimental colorectal carcinogenesis. Anticancer Res 9:1477–1482

Nelson RL, Davis FG, Satter E, Sobin LH, Kikendall W, Bowen P (1994) Body iron stores and risk of colonic neoplasia. J Natl Cancer Inst 86:455–460

Newmark HL, Wargovich MJ, Bruce WR (1984) Colon cancer and dietary fat, phosphate and calcium: a hypothesis. J Natl Cancer Inst 72:1323–1325

Nielson BK, Thompson LU, Bird RP (1987) Effect of phytic acid on colonic cell proliferation. Cancer Lett 37:317–325

O'Neil GP, Ford Hutchinson AW (1993) Expression of mRNA for cyclooxygenase-1 and cyclooxygenase-2 in human tissues. FEBS Lett 330:156–160

Owen RW, Weisgerber UM, Carr J, Harrison MH (1995) The analysis of calcium-lipid complexes in faeces. Eur J Cancer Prev 4:247–255

Owen RW, Weisgerber UM, Spiegelhalder B, Bartsch H (1996a) Faecal phytic acid and its relation to other putative markers of risk for colorectal cancer. Gut 38:591–597

Owen RW, Wimonwatwatee T, Spiegelhalder B, Bartsch H (1996b) A high performance liquid chromatography system for quantification of hydroxyl radical formation by determination of dihydroxy benzoic acids. Eur J Cancer Prev 5:233–240

Paganini-Hill A (1994) Aspirin and the prevention of colorectal cancer: a review of the evidence. Semin Surg Oncol 10:158–164

Rafter JJ, Eng VWS, Furrer R, Medline A, Bruce WR (1986) Effects of calcium and pH on the mucosal damage produced by deoxycholic acid in the rat colon. Gut 27:1320–1329

Reddy BS, Wynder EL (1973) Etiology of cancer of the colon. J Natl Cancer Inst 50:1437–1442

Reddy BS, Wynder EL (1977) Metabolic epidemiology of colon cancer: fecal bile acids and neutral sterols in colon cancer patients and patients with adenomatous polyps. Cancer 39:2533–2539

Rozen P, Fireman Z, Fine N, Wax Y, Ron E (1989) Oral calcium suppresses increased rectal proliferation of persons at risk of colorectal cancer. Gut 30:650–655

Risio M, Lipkin M, Candelaresi G, Bertone A, Coverlizza S, Rossini FP (1991) Correlations between rectal mucosa cell proliferation and the clinical and pathological features of nonfamilial neoplasia of the large intestine. Cancer Res 51:1917–1921

Silverman SJ, Andrews AW (1977) Bile acids: co-mutagenic activity in the salmonella-mammalian microsome mutagenicity test. J Natl Cancer Inst 59:1557–1559

Sorenson AW, Slattery ML, Ford MH (1988) Calcium and colon cancer: a review. Nutr Cancer 11:135–145

Steinbach G, Lupton J, Reddy BS, Kral JG, Holt PR (1994) Effect of calcium supplementation on rectal epithelial hyperproliferation in intestinal bypass subjects. Gastroenterology 106:1162–1167

Stern HS, Gregoire RC, Kashtan H, Stadler J, Bruce WR (1990) Long-term effects of dietary calcium on risk markers for colon cancer in patients with familial polyposis. Surgery 108:528–533

Stevens RG, Jones DY, Micozzi MS, Taylor PR (1988) Body iron stores and risk for cancer. N Engl J Med 319:1047–1052

Ullah A, Shamsuddin AM (1990) Dose-dependent inhibition of large intestinal cancer by inositol hexaphosphate in F344 rats. Carcinogenesis 11:2219-2222

Van der Meer R, De Vries HT (1985) Differential binding of glycine- and taurine-conjugated bile acids to insoluble calcium phosphate. Biochem J 229:265-268

Van der Meer R, Welberg JWM, Kuipers F, Kleibeuker JH, Mulder NH, Termont DSML, Vonk RJ, De Vries HT, De Vries EGE (1990) Effects of supplementary dietary calcium on the intestinal association of calcium, phosphate and bile acids. Gastroenterology 99:1653-1659

Waddell WR, Loughry RW (1983) Sulindac for polyposis of the colon. J Surg Oncol 24:83-87

Wargovich MJ, Eng VWS, Newmark HL, Bruce WR (1983) Calcium ameliorates the toxic effect of deoxycholic acid on colonic epithelium. Carcinogenesis 4:1205-1207

Wargovich MJ, Eng VWS, Newmark HL (1984) Calcium inhibits the damaging and compensatory proliferation effects of fatty acids on mouse colon epithelium. Cancer Lett 23:253-258

Welberg JWM, Kleibeuker JH, Van der Meer R, Kuipers F, Cats A, Van-Rijsbergen H, Termont DSML, Boersma Van EW, Vonk RJ, Mulder NH, De Vries EGE (1993) Effects of oral calcium supplementation on intestinal bile acids and cytolytic activity of fecal water in patients with adenomatous polyps of the colon. Eur J Clin Invest 23:63-68

Weisgerber UM, Boeing H, Owen RW, Raedsch R, Wahrendorf J (1996) Effect of long-term placebo-controlled calcium supplementation on sigmoidal cell proliferation in patients with sporadic adenomatotous polyps. Gut 38:396-402

Whitfield JF (1992) Calcium signals and cancer. Crit Rev Oncol 3:55-90

Willett WC, Stampfer MJ, Colditz GA, Rosner BA, Speizer FE (1990) Relation of meat, fat and fiber intake to the risk of colon cancer in a prospective study among women. N Engl J Med 323:1664-1672

Wilpart M, Mainguet P, Maskens A, Roberfroid M (1983) Mutagenicity of 1,2-dimethylhydrazine towards *Salmonella typhimurium*: co-mutagenic effect of secondary bile acids. Carcinogenesis 6:45-48

Winde G, Schmid KW, Schlegel W, Fischer R, Osswald H, Bünte H (1995) Complete reversion and prevention of rectal adenomas in colectomized patients with familial adenomatous polyposis by rectal low-dose sulindac maintenance therapy. Dis Colon Rectum 38:813-830

Diagnosis and Therapeutic Relevance of Micrometastases

E. Holz[1], K. Pantel[2], and G. Riethmüller[2]

[1] Munich Tumor Center, Faculty of Medicine, Ludwig-Maximilians University and Technical University, Maistrasse 11, 80337 Munich, Germany
[2] Institute of Immunology University of Munich, Goethestrasse 31, 80336 Munich, Germany

Abstract

The disseminated isolated tumor cell has become a formidable object of solid tumor research for at least three good reasons: it can be identified in organ compartments such as bone marrow, blood, and lymph nodes and, once found, it can be morphologically characterized with respect to tumor-associated antigens, oncogenes, tumor suppressor genes, proliferation markers, and/or growth receptors. Thirdly, it is also an ideal target for immunotherapy directed at accessible, well-defined membrane-associated antigens of the tumor cell.

Diagnostic Relevance of Micrometastases

The disseminated isolated tumor cell can be diagnosed using immunocytochemical techniques. The prognostic impact of disseminated tumor cells has been well established over the past 10 years by correlating the immunocytochemical finding of disseminated tumor cells in secondary organs such as the bone marrow and lymph nodes with disease-free survival of patients (Table 1). In addition, its phenotype can be further characterized by double marker analysis. Information on the phenotype of early disseminated carci-

Table 1. Detection and prognostic significance of micrometastatic tumor cells in patients with epithelial cancers

Secondary organ	Tumor origin	Marker	Published report on prognostic value
Bone marrow	Breast	EMA	Mansi et al. (1991)
		Cytokeratin	Schlimok et al. (1992)
		TAG 12	Diel et al. (1992)
	Colorectum	Cytokeratin	Lindemann et al. (1992)
	Stomach	Cytokeratin	Schlimok et al. (1991)
	Lung (NSCLC)	Cytokeratin	Pantel et al. (1993a)
Lymph nodes	Breast	Cytokeratin	De Mascarel et al. (1992)
	Lung	BerEp4	Passlick et al. (1994)

EMA, epithelial membrane antigen; TAG 12 tumor antigen 12; NSCLC, non-small-cell lung cancer.

Table 2. Characterization of micrometastatic tumor cells in bone marrow

Marker	Tumor origin	Number of patients with marker +/CK+ cells		Reference
		n/toal	%	
Tumor-associated antigens				
17-1A	Breast	7/16	43.8	Pantel & Riethmüller (1994)
	Colorectum	4/6	66.7	Pantel & Riethmüller (1994)
Growth factor receptors				
EGF-R	Breast	10/37	27.0	Schlimok & Riethmüller (1990)
	Colorectum	4/15	26.7	Schlimok & Riethmüller (1990)
erbB2	Breast	48/71	67.6	Pantel et al. (1993b)
	Colorectum/stomach	14/50	28.0	Pantel et al. (1993b)
MHC class I antigen				
	Breast	9/26	34.6	Pantel et al. (1991)
	Colon/stomach	37/65	56.9	Pantel et al. (1991)
Adhesion molecules				
ICAM1	Lung (NSCLC)	13/31	41.9	Pantel et al. (1992)
Proliferation-associated proteins				
Ki-67	Breast	1/12	8.3	Pantel et al. (1993b)
	Colorectum/stomach	0/21	0	Pantel et al. (1993b)
p120	Breast	1/11	9.1	Pantel et al. (1993b)
	Colorectum/stomach	9/32	28.1	Pantel et al. (1993b)

noma cells may aid in defining the right strategy in treating individual cancer patients. For example, proliferation-associated antigens such as Ki-67 or p 120 are present in less than 30% of Cytokeratin (CK)-positive cells, indicating that these tumor cells are in G_0 phase.

Growth factor receptors such as erbB2 are expressed in up to 68% of CK-positive cells in breast cancer patients, indicating that this molecule may be a relevant target for therapy of breast cancer patients. Similarly, the tumor-associated antigen 17-1A is expressed in 67% of CK-positive cells in colorectal cancer patients and may thus represent a target for therapeutic strategies (Table 2).

Therapeutic Relevance of Micrometastases

The disseminated tumor cell is an easily accessible and vulnerable target for minimal residual cancer therapy. Here, two examples of successful immunotherapy directed at these tumor cells are given. In a recently published pharmacodynamic study (Schlimok et al. 1995), patients with breast and colorectal cancer presenting with CK-positive tumor cells in bone marrow were randomized to treatment either with six infusions of 100 mg each of a Lewis

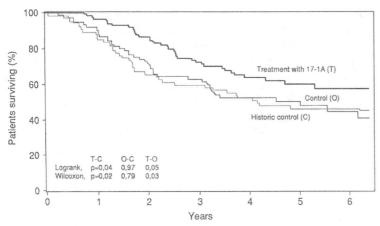

Fig. 1. Overall survival in patients with colorectal cancer: effect of antibody therapy (17-1A) after surgery. Historic controls are a group of patients from Hanover

Y monoclonal antibody or to six infusions of placebo consisting of human serum albumin (HSA) during a 2-week treatment period. CK-positive cells in marrow were monitored prior to and after treatment with the underlying hypothesis that treatment might reduce the number of cells. Evaluable quantitative data were obtained in 10 breast cancer patients presenting with more than 20 tumor cells per 4×10^5 nucleated bone marrow cells at baseline. Of seven patients randomized to the antibody arm, five showed eradication or a distinct reduction of CK-positive/Lewis Y-positive cells, defined as reduction of at least one log unit or to zero cells. On the other hand, two patients presenting with Lewis Y-negative tumor cells and all three patients who received the placebo infusion showed no corresponding decrease of tumor cells. The authors postulate that the reduction of isolated tumor cells carrying the Lewis Y antigen was due to the cytotoxic action of the injected Lewis Y monoclonal antibody. This trial indicates that expression of the relevant target antigen structure on the isolated tumor cell and the specifically directed cytotoxic agent are pertinent to obtaining efficacious results.

Another target system is defined by the 17-1A antibody (Koprowski et al. 1979) which recognizes a 37 to 40-Kda glycoprotein expressed on the cell surface of a wide variety of epithelial tumors (Göttlinger et al. 1986). The function of the 17-1A antigen has been claimed to be related to cell–cell adhesion of epithelial cells (Litvinov et al. 1994). As it is highly conserved throughout evolution, it may have indeed an important function in epithelial cell physiology (Velders et al. 1994). The 17-1A antibody was put to a more rigidly controlled test of clinical efficacy by infusing it into patients with high-risk colorectal cancer after complete resection of their primary tumor (Riethmüller et al. 1994) and measuring clinical endpoints such as disease-free and overall survival. In this adjuvant trial, patients were randomized to receive either a total of 900 mg mAb 17-1A in five infusions over 20 weeks starting at 2–3 weeks after surgery or to no further treatment. After a median follow-up of 5 years, antibody therapy reduced the overall death rate by 30% and decreased the recurrence rate by 27% (Fig. 1). It is noteworthy that the therapeutic effect was most pronounced on the prevention of distant metastases as site of first recurrence after surgery (p <0.004), supporting the hypothesis that the isolated tumor cell, generally believed to be the originator of later distant relapse, is the primary target of immunotherapy. The results of this trial are similar to those reported for (radio)chemotherapy with regard to efficacy (Moertel et al. 1990; Krook et al. 1991). However, the toxicity observed after 17-1A treatment is considerably lower (Riethmüller et al. 1994).

Implications of Micrometastases for Disease Management

The above data also demonstrate the limitations of any form of adjuvant therapy applied to all patients with a particular disease in a particular stage. In regard to stage III colorectal cancer, only 15 of 100 patients treated will benefit from any adjuvant therapy following surgery, which should lead to two conclusions: as long as it is unknown which patients may benefit from therapy, the least toxic regimen at equal efficacy should be employed to minimize risk to the 85 of 100 patients who will not benefit. Secondly, more efforts need to be applied to searching out a priori those patients at higher risk of relapse, so that eventually only patients at higher risk will receive further custome-tailored or -specific adjuvant therapy.

The demonstration of isolated tumor cells at sites distant from the primary tumor may in future become a critical test for the decision whether further therapy is warranted. Furthermore, characterization of these cells may give additional clues as to which therapeutic modality may be most suitable and beneficial for the individual patient.

References

De Mascarel I, Bonichon F, Coindre JM, Trojani-M (1992) Prognostic significance of breast cancer axillary lymph node micrometastases assessed by two special techniques: reevaluation with longer follow-up. Br J Cancer 66:523–527

Diel IJ, Kaufmann M, Goerner R, Costa SD, Kaul S, Bastert G (1992) Detection of tumor cells in bone marrow of patients with primary breast cancer: a prognostic factor for distant metastasis. J Clin Oncol 10:1534–1539

Göttlinger HG, Funke I, Johnson JP, Gokel JM, Riethmüller G (1986) The epithelial cell surface antigen 17-1A, a target for antibody-mediated tumor therapy: its biochemical nature, tissue distribution and recognition by different monoclonal antibodies. Int J Cancer 38:47–53

Koprowski H, Steplewski Z, Mitchell K et al (1979) Colorectal carcinoma antigens detected by hybridoma antibodies. Somat Cell Genet 5:957–972

Krook JE, Moertel CG, Gunderson LL, Wieand HS, Collins RT, Beart RW, Kubista TP, Poon MA, Meyers WC, Mailliard JA et al (1991) Effective surgical adjuvant therapy for high-risk rectal carcinoma. N Engl J Med 324:709–715

Lindemann F, Schlimok G, Dirschedl P, Witte J, Riethmüller G (1992) Prognostic significance of micrometastatic tumor cells in bone marrow of colorectal cancer patients. Lancet 340:685-689

Litvinov SV, Velders MP, Bakker HA, Fleuren GJ, Warnaar SO (1994) Ep-CAM: a human epithelial antigen is a homophilic cell-cell adhesion molecule. J Cell Biol 125:437-446

Mansi JL, Easton D, Berger U, Gazet JC, Ford HT, Dearnaley D, Coombes RC (1991) Bone marrow micrometastases in primary breast cancer: prognostic significance after 6 years follow-up. Eur J Cancer 27:1552-1555

Moertel CG, Fleming TR, MacDonald JS, Haller DG, Laurie JA, Goodman PJ, Ungerleider JS, Emerson WA, Tormey DC, Glick JH et al (1990) Levamisole and fluorouracil for adjuvant therapy of resected colon carcinoma. N Engl J Med 322:352-358.

Pantel K, Riethmüller G (1994) Detection, characterization and antibody therapy of minimal residual epithelial cancer. Oncol Today 11:4-9

Pantel K, Schlimok G, Kutter D, Schaller G, Genz T, Wiebecke B, Backmann R, Funke I, Riethmüller G (1991) Frequent down regulation of major histocompatibility class I antigen expression on individual micrometastatic carcinoma cells. Cancer Res 51:4712-4715

Pantel K, Angstwurm M, Kutter D et al (1992) Down-regulation and neo-expression of cell surface antigens on individual micrometastatic carcinoma cells. Contrib Oncol 44:283-293

Pantel K, Izbicki JR, Angstwurm M, Braun S, Passlick B, Karg O, Thetter O, Riethmüller G (1993a) Immunocytological detection of bone marrow micrometastasis in operable non-small cell lung cancer. Cancer Res 53:1027-1031

Pantel K, Schlimok G, Braun S, Kutter D, Lindemann F, Schaller G, Funke I, Izbicki JR, Riethmüller G (1993b) Differential expression of proliferation-associated molecules in individual micrometastatic carcinoma cells, J Natl Cancer Inst 85:1419-1424

Passlick B, Izbick JR, Kubuschok B, Nathrath W, Thetter O, Pichlmeier U, Schweiberer L, Riethmüller G, Pantel K (1994) Immunohistochemical assessment of individual tumor cells in lymph nodes of patients with non-small cell lung cancer. J Clin Oncol 12:1827-1823

Riethmüller G, Schneider-Gädicke E, Schlimok G, Schmiegel W, Raab R, Höffken K, Gruber R, Pichlmaier H, Hirche H, Pichlmayr R et al (1994) Randomized trial of monoclonal antibody for adjuvant therapy of resected Dukes's C colorectal carcinoma, Lancet 343:1177-1183

Schlimok G, Riethmüller G (1990) Detection, characterization and tumorigenicity of disseminated tumor cells in human bone marrow. Semin Cancer Biol 1:207-215

Schlimok G, Funke I, Pantel K, Strobel F, Lindemann F, Witte J, Riethmüller G (1991) Micrometastatic tumor cells in bone marrow of patients with gastric cancer: methodological aspects of detection and prognostic significance. Eur J Cancer 27:1461-1465

Schlimok G, Lindemann F, Holzmann K et al (1992) Prognostic significance of disseminated tumor cells detected in bone marrow of patients with breast and colorectal cancer: a multivariate analysis. Proc ASCO 11:102 (abstr)

Schlimok G, Pantel K, Loibner H, Fackler-Schwalbe I, Riethmüller G (1995) Reduction of metastasic carcinoma cells in bone marrow by intravenously administered monoclonal antibody: towards a novel surrogate test to monitor adjuvant therapies of solid tumors. Eur J Cancer 31 A, 11:1799-1803

Velders MP, Litvinov SV, Warnaar SO, Gorter A, Fleuren GJ, Zurawski VR Jr, Coney LR (1994) New chimeric antipancarcinoma monoclonal antibody with superior cytotoxicity-mediating potency. Cancer Res 54:1753-1759

Subject Index

A
17-1A 215
Abdominal perineal excision 59, 88, 95, 101, 114, 122, 150
Abdominoperineal resection 105 f., 112
Adenoma 20, 23, 200
Adenomatous polyposis coli 12
Adhesion molecules 214 f.
Adjuvant radiotherapy 148
– therapy 111, 141, 159, 217
Alcohol 204
Amsterdam criterias 22
Anal competence 172
– sphincter 60, 110
Aneuploidy 7
Angiography 134
Anorectal reconstruction 105, 112
Anterior rectal resection 44, 59, 87, 136
Antibody therapy 215
Anti-inflammatory drugs 203
APC gene 12, 50
Aspirin 203, 210
Autosomal dominant inheritance pattern 21

B
Bile acids 196
Biofeedback 100
Bone marrow 215
Breast cancer 28
BSD-2000 system 175 ff.

C
Calcium 196
Cancer family 20, 29
CEA 49 ff.
Cell proliferation 142, 197
– spillage 127, 132
Chemoprevention 195, 200, 210
Chemotherapy 96, 153, 159

Coloanal anastomosis 87, 161 ff.,
Colonic pouch 89, 91, 93, 99, 110
– reservoir 88
Colonoscopy 23
Colorectal adenomas 20, 23, 200, 203
– anastomosis 109
Colostomy 64, 95, 99, 108
Combined modality approach 153
– – therapy 133
Comparative genomic hybridization 5, 8
Continent urinary reservoirs 76
Cytokeratin 214 f.
Cytostatic drug resistance 14

D
Deleted in colon cancer genes 13
Denonvilier's fascia 68
Dietary factors 24, 210
– fibre 195
DNA-based diagnosis 23
– cytophotometry 7
– mismatch repair genes 20, 22
– testing 23
Downstaging 175 ff.
Dysplasia 5

E
EGF-R 215
Electromanometry 106
Electromyostimulation 105, 107 f, 112
Endoluminal ultrasound 106, 134
Endometric cancer 21
Endorectal MRI 36, 41 ff.
– ultrasound 44, 150, 175 ff.
Endosonography 89, 121
erbB2 215
Exenteration 73 ff., 79
Exenterative surgery 73
Extensive surgery 59
Extenterative pelvic operations 72

Extracolonic malignancies   21

F
FAP   12, 49 f., 204 f.
Fascia of Gerota   67
Fecal blood tests   49
– continence   63 f., 95
– incontinence   92, 101, 105, 109 f.
5-Fluorouracil   145, 156, 159
5-FU   145, 159
Fluorescence in situ hybridization   5
Full-thickness resection   117

G
Genetic alterations   9, 20, 51
Genitourinary morbidity   132
Genotype   3
Glass specula   115
Gluteus myocutaneous flaps   76
Gracilis neosphincter   105
Graciloplasty   76, 102, 107
Gynaecological screening   23

H
Hereditary nonpolyposis colorectal cancer   21, 49, 20 ff.
High-dose external irradiation   161 ff.
hMLH1 gene   22
hMLH2 gene   26
HNPCC   49 f., 20 ff.
HNPCC registries   29
Hyperthermia   175 ff.
Hyperthermic radiochemotherapy   96
Hypogastric nerves   66

I
Immunotherapy   142
Implantable devices   108
Implantation metastases   131, 132
In situ hybridization   5
Inferior hypogastric plexus   68
– mesenteric artery   134
Infrarectal space   69
Intersphincteric resection   62, 64, 89
Interval cancer   23
Intraoperative radiotherapy   154 ff., 176
Irradiated pelvis   75

J
Jejunal conduit   76

K
K-ras mutation   49, 53

L
Lage bowel cancer   25

Late severe colitis   153
– toxicity   152
Leucovorin   156
Local excision   114 ff.
– recurrence   52, 62, 88, 109, 119 ff., 127, 132, 136, 142 f.
– tumor control   152
Locoregional recurrence   128
Loss of heterozygosity   5
Low anterior resection   61
Lymph node   6, 43, 61
– – involvement   9
– – metastases   121, 128
Lynch syndromes   22

M
Mesorectal excision   66, 97, 136, 87
Mesorectum   60, 135
Methyl-CCNU   145
MHC   215
MIB-1   7
Micrometastases   7, 215
Microsatellite instability   22
Molecular genetic   49
– pathology   4
Monoclonal antibodies   214 f.
Morbidity   77, 156
Mortality   77, 210
MRI imaging   36 ff.
Multidrug resistance   14
Multimodal therapy   175 ff.
Multimodality approach   160
Mutated in colorectal cancer genes   12
Mutation   49
Mutator genes   13

N
Neorectal compliance   64
Neosphincter   95 ff.
Nerve-sparing surgery   132
NME1/Nm23-H1   11
NME2/Nm23-H2   11
No-touch isolation technique   137

O
Operative mortality   79

P
p 53   10, 53
Parietal pelvic fascia   67
Pain   80
PCR   49
Pedicled omental plug   77
Pelvic dead space   76
– exenteration   72, 80
– urinary enteric conduit   77

Subject Index

Pelvirectal fibrous space 67
Penetrance 21
Perineal colostomy 111
- fistulae 81
- wound 76
Perineural invasion 131
Perioperative management 172
Peritoneal cytology 131
Phenotype 3
Physiotherapy 99
Phytic acid 200, 210
Polyps 204
Post-exenteration prognosis 78
- quality of life 81
- relapse 78
Posterior exenteration 75
Postoperative irradiation 144
- radiotherapy 63, 141, 146 f., 150
Pouch 87
Preoperative external radiation 174
- radio-chemo-thermotherapy 175 ff.
- radiotherapy 62, 141, 144
- staging 110
Prerectal fibrous space 68
Presymptomatic DNA testing 23
Prognostic factors 6, 49 f., 122
Proliferation index 198
Prophylactic colectomy 24
Prophylactic hysterectomy 23
Psychosocial sequelae 26

Q
Quality of life 80, 111, 162

R
R0 resection 118, 122
Radiation schedule 145
Radiation enteritis 75
- therapy 122
Radiochemotherapy 102, 141, 153, 175 ff., 217
Radiotherapy 131, 146, 149, 175 ff.
RAS Gene Family 10
Reactive oxygen 206
Rectal adenoma 40
- excision 91
Retosacral fascia 68
Rectotomy 62

Rectus abdominis 76
Recurrence 51, 62, 72, 78, 173, 217
Regional hyperthermia 175 ff.
Replication-error 22
Residual disease 159
Response 175 ff.

S
Screening 49
Seromuscular sphincter 101
Sigmoid colon conduits 76
Single-strand conformation
  polymorphism 5
Sphincter function 61, 63, 141
- preservation 161
- - resection 88
- - preservation surgery 161 ff.
- sparing procedures 60
Squeeze pressure 63
Sulindac 204, 210
Superior hypogastric plexus 68
Survival 78, 120, 145, 176
Suture material 129

T
Target volume 156
TATA 162 f., 172, 174
Telomerase 15
Tensor fascia lata 76
Total pelvic exenteration 72
Transanal excision 61, 141
Tumor associated antigens 214 ff.
- biology 59
- proliferation 142
- - spillage 127
- markers 48

U
Ultrasonography 44
Uretersigmoidostomy 76
Urinary diversion 76, 78

V
Vaginal reconstruction 77
Vitamin E 204

W
Waldeyer's fascia 68